EMERGENCY 24/7:

NURSES OF THE EMERGENCY ROOM

ECHO HERON

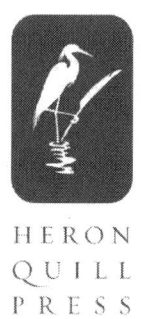

HERON
QUILL
PRESS

ALSO BY ECHO HERON

Nonfiction

INTENSIVE CARE: The Story of a Nurse

CONDITION CRITICAL: The Story of a Nurse Continues

TENDING LIVES: Nurses on the Medical Front

Fiction

MERCY

NOON AT TIFFANY'S (historical, biographical novel)

Mysteries

The Adele Monsarrat series:

PULSE

PANIC

PARADOX

FATAL DIAGNOSIS

Copyright © 2015 by Echo Heron

All rights reserved

No part of this book may be reproduced in any form or by any electronic or mechanical means including information storage and retrieval systems without permission in writing from the author. The only exception is by a reviewer, who may quote short excerpts in a review.

Published in the United States by Heron Quill Press, LLC

EMERGENCY 24/7:

Nurses of the Emergency Room

http:/www.echoheron.com

ISBN: 978-1-938439-67-4

Nursing—Anecdotes

Cover design: Aldren Gamalo

Formatting: Polgarus Studio

Interior design: Rachael Garrity, PenWorthy, LLC

Author photo: Steven Vermillion

This book is meant to describe the experiences, thoughts and feelings of emergency room nurses, including nurses who worked directly with the victims of the September 11, 2001 attacks. The chapters herein are based on taped interviews with these nurses. The scenes contained in this book are based on real life events that the contributors have described to me.

With the exception of ten of the eleven September 11, 2001 nurses and the Ebola Treatment Center nurse who agreed to the use of their actual names, titles, and locations, I have used fictitious names and physical characteristics for all other nurses, patients, family members, doctors, auxiliary healthcare providers, hospitals, and institutions portrayed herein. In some cases, I have also altered the chronology and place of events. I must do this due to legal requirements for protection of both nurse and patient confidentiality. This book is not meant to focus criticism on any particular group, institution, or individual. Any resemblances the reader may imagine they discern are unintended and entirely coincidental.

The views and opinions expressed by the individuals featured in this book do not necessarily reflect those of the author.

As always—for the nurses

CONTENTS

AUTHOR'S NOTE	iii
CASSIE	1
SUZANNE PUGH,	
St. Vincent's, NYC	8
FAYE	21
MOLLY	30
ANN CARROLL,	
Ground Zero, NYC	37
KIT	48
NORMA	62
KATHLEEN HOLLOWED,	
Washington Hospital Burn Center	86
JILL	93
GLORIA	108
NANCY ISSING,	
St. Vincent's, NYC	117
JESSICA	128
APRIL	133
LORRAINE ENSMINGER,	
Beth Israel, NYC	146
STELLA	162
LUCILLE YIP,	
St. Vincent's, NYC	168
ROBIN	182
OLGA	190
ANGEL LOPEZ,	
Ground Zero, NYC	192
DARCY	200
WANDA	209

PETER ALLAR,
    St. Vincent's, NYC 214
MAGGIE 224
CLEO 241
BOB DEMBIKI,
    Cornell Burn Center, NYC 245
MARIAH 250
DANIEL 256
JAY CIVELLO,
    St. Vincent's, NYC 261
MICK 269
ANONYMOUS,
    Ground Zero, NYC 272
SUE AVERILL,
    Ebola Treatment Center, Africa 279
AFTERWORD 293
ACKNOWLEDGMENTS 295

Author's Note

Emergency 24/7: Nurses of the Emergency Room is based on recorded interviews I conducted with emergency room nurses from all parts of the United States. I had just finished these interviews and was fashioning them into chapters, when September 11, 2001 changed our lives forever. At my agent's suggestion, I interviewed a number of nurses who worked in New York City and Washington D.C. that day and in the weeks to follow.

In the spring of 2002, *Emergency 24/7* was sent to various publishers. The collective response was that it was too soon after 9/11, and that the public—still emotionally raw from the catastrophic event—was not ready for these stories.

Since I personally conducted these highly sensitive and emotional interviews, I understood this sentiment—to a degree. Except, as I looked around, I saw a profusion of 9/11 books being published, most of which focused on the experiences of the paramedics, policemen and firemen. Why, I wondered, among these many stories of tragedy, heroism and courage, was there no room for a book in which the voices of the nurses might be heard?

Two years later, we again tried to interest editors in *Emergency 24/7*. This time, the rejections were largely based on the opinion that the narratives were too haunting and too emotionally charged. Again, I found many true medicine books and articles that were just as haunting, and emotionally charged.

A year later, I tried once more to interest publishers in this book. This time I received a straightforward, though somewhat misguided, set of responses. The one that best summed up the general attitude was, "No one is interested in reading about nurses. If your interviews were with doctors, firemen or paramedics, we would be much more willing to take on this book."

At that point, my agent advised me to put the book away and forget about it. I did put the book away—but I could not forget about it. In 2014 I dusted off the manuscript and decided it was finally time to let the nurses' voices be heard.

Echo Heron
San Francisco, 2015

CASSIE

"Did everybody's grandmother die last year and now no one on earth knows about the old-fashioned common sense remedies like warm saltwater gargles for sore throats, and ice for bruises and sprains? Has everyone gone mad with the obsession that they MUST see a doctor NOW? A child burps and the parents rush him to ER. A twenty-year-old gets a headache, and she calls for an ambulance.

"I have come to the conclusion that no one has to fire a shot to take over America—all they have to do is release a cold virus. This society is incapable of dealing with the littlest owie."

I don't know who the twit was who designed our ER, but whoever they were, I'd be willing to bet they'd never been in one—it is a certainty they'd never worked in one.

Our glass-fronted treatment rooms are set up along both sides of the main corridor of the ambulance intake bay. Three trauma rooms are situated at the opposite end of that corridor. This means that when a rig pulls in, all the patients in those cubicles can see and hear the pandemonium that goes on around the stretcher as it progresses from the ambulance bay doors to the trauma rooms.

We always warn the patients, "If an ambulance comes in and you can't handle seeing horrible things—don't look." Some heed that warning, others don't. I've seen grown men break down in tears, throw up and pass out at the sight of what sometimes come in on those stretchers.

It was springtime, when people were venturing out of their caves and engaging in sports, home repairs and gardening. We'd been steadily busy all day with lacerations, sprained ankles and eye injuries. The treatment rooms were never empty. As soon as one patient would leave, the sheet was replaced and another patient would come in.

When the radio shrieked a code three alarm, we ran for the main trauma room. A code three alarm was rare. It meant a big hairy trauma was coming our way and we needed to pull out all the stops. We moved like greased lightening around the trauma room, opening the crash cart, setting up suction and stocking in numerous bags of intravenous solutions. The OR, anesthesia, and the blood bank were put on red alert.

As we worked, the paramedics radioed in their ETA and said there'd been a drive-by shooting in a middle-class residential neighborhood. Because the victim was bleeding out from multiple gunshot wounds, they'd done a load-and-go rather than stabilize him in the field. CPR was in progress, an endotracheal tube was in place, and two large-bore intravenous lines had been inserted.

In the paramedic's voice I heard something that sounded like horror, shock, and grief—rare qualities to hear in the voice of a seasoned paramedic.

I ran outside to meet the rig and out of the corner of my eye, I noticed a Jeep parked at an extreme angle next to the ambulance. The Jeep's motor was still running and the driver's door stood open, but no one was behind the wheel.

Through the narrow windows of the ambulance's back doors, I caught a glimpse of a paramedic hunched over the patient, his back moving in rhythm to the CPR polka. Outside, frantically pummeling the doors was a woman in the advanced stages of pregnancy. She was screaming, her words incomprehensible.

She stumbled back when the doors of the rig slammed open and the paramedics backed out, pulling the stretcher with them.

My eyes automatically went to the patient. I got a brief look at a masculine jaw, but the finer features of the man's face were obscured by a massive amount of blood. The paramedic straddling the man continued doing CPR without looking up.

The pregnant woman rushed the gurney, but the ambulance driver caught her and, with some effort, pulled her away. In the light, her skin was so pale, that for a second I wondered if she'd been injured as well.

I ran alongside the gurney, trying to block out the sound of the woman screaming her husband's name. The driver put his arms around her and held her firmly while he spoke into her ear. Whatever he was saying seemed to calm her, for she stopped screaming and let him lead her toward the main entrance.

"Thirty-seven-year-old male was working in the front yard while his six-year-old daughter played nearby," reported the paramedic pushing the stretcher. "The next door neighbor said he saw the car drive by with some kind of automatic weapon mounted in the rear passenger window. He shouted a warning, but the gun was already firing.

"The six-year-old took five hits to the neck and head. She was dead at the scene. Dad caught fire in the abdomen, chest and neck. He looked so bad when we got there, we just did a load and go. He knew his name and asked about his daughter, but by the time we got him into the rig, he was nonresponsive without blood pressure or rhythm.

"The wife was at the back of the house. She thought someone was shooting off firecrackers. When she got to the front of the house a minute later, the car was gone."

As we ran past the treatment rooms, I saw the looks of horror on the waiting patients' faces. Some turned away, some covered their eyes. No one could complain that they weren't getting a show worth the wait.

I was already thinking in terms of what actions to take and what drugs to give, when my mind registered a tiny, peculiar blip. It was like walking into a familiar, well-ordered room and instinctively knowing that something is out of place or missing.

My eyes darted back to treatment room fifteen, presently occupied by a soccer mom and her ten-year-old son who'd come in complaining of a sore throat. Both mom and son leaned casually against the wall, arms crossed, watching the approaching train wreck with bored indifference.

I searched their faces for some tiny seed of human emotion, but found nothing gentle or even surprised. Their expressions were in such perverse contrast to what was going on in front of them that I blinked to make sure I was seeing clearly.

The crisis taking place in the trauma room drove the small observation from my mind as the ten of us feverishly worked to keep the man from bleeding to death.

The ER doctor was trying to get another large bore IV into the patient while the surgeon cracked the man's chest and did cardiac massage with his gloved hand inside the chest cavity. The rest of us were silent, waiting for some sign of hope.

I had just made note of how tired everyone looked, when several of the nurses' expressions change to wide-eyed astonishment.

I turned around slowly, fully expecting to see a gang member with a gun. Instead, I came face to face with the soccer mom from treatment room fifteen. I was rendered speechless. Never in my memory had a layperson unrelated to the patient had the gall to enter the closed doors of a trauma room where a code was in full progress.

Soccer mom tugged at my arm. "I need to speak with you outside for a moment." Her eyes didn't so much as flicker toward the man dying on the table less than ten inches away.

I hustled her out into the hallway where she tapped the crystal of her expensive watch. "We've been waiting here for over an hour and a half. How much longer is that going to take in there? My son is uncomfortable and he has to be at lacrosse practice in a half-hour. Can't one of those doctors pop out for a few minutes to see him?" She made a noise of exasperation. "I mean really, how many doctors and nurses can one person require?"

I opened my mouth, and then shut it long enough to get control of myself. "There's a man dying in there," I said at last. "He needs all the personnel we can spare him."

"So, does that mean the rest of us have to suffer?" A touch of sarcasm laced her voice.

I stared at her trying to understand what happened to people like this that caused them to be so insensitive and devoid of empathy. In disgust I turned away and left her standing in the hall.

I returned to the fray still going on in the trauma room. The code lasted another few minutes then it was over. None of us could speak. Emotionally, we were all shell-shocked.

I was given the task of bringing the wife to the Privacy Room, which was where we told the survivors of their loss. More often than not, the emotional carnage that took place in the Privacy Room was a hundred times worse than the blood and gore in the trauma rooms.

I found the widow, who didn't know she was a widow yet, in the chaplain's office, absently running her hands over her pregnant belly. She was now silent and docile, deep inside that shocked foggy state that often surrounds the survivors. I told her she needed to come with me and gently put my arm around her waist, lifting her to her feet. She leaned into me, letting her head rest on my shoulder. The small, intimate gesture made my heart ache. I half carried her, feeling as though I was leading her to her death. More than anything I wanted to protect her from the news that awaited her.

Unfortunately, the only way to get to the Privacy Room is to pass down the hall of treatment rooms. We were a few feet from our destination, when soccer mom stepped in front of us, blocking our way. Her fury was visible.

"*Now* do you think we can get someone in here to see my son, or is everyone going to take a coffee break?"

I pushed past her without answering, but the widow took soccer mom's hand in hers and studied her face. "I am so sorry," she whispered in the soft voice the walking wounded use while still in shock. "My little girl was killed today. She was only six. The doctors and nurses are trying to save my husband. I'm sorry about your son. I wish I could help, but I can't because . . . because . . ."

Soccer mom pulled her hand away and stepped aside, her expression one of utter contempt, as if the woman's tragedy might be contagious.

The widow and I moved on to the Privacy Room where one of the doctors was waiting to break the news. I stayed with her until her sister arrived.

By the time I was able to leave the small massacre that had taken place in the Privacy Room, soccer mom and son were gone.

I sometimes wonder what soccer mom thought of that small brush with raw reality. I wonder too, if in one of her more human moments, she might comprehend what the pregnant widow was feeling, and find within herself some trace of compassion.

Who knows? Maybe she'll never think of it at all.

SUZANNE PUGH
St. Vincent's Hospital, ER nurse manager
New York City resident

"Let me put it to you this way, my sister sends me this nice little notebook so I could journal everything that happened to me that day, right? Yeah, well, it's still blank.

"My boyfriend says, 'Suzanne, you've got to do what Oprah talks about—journaling.'

"I say, 'Honey, you watch too much daytime TV, and since when did journaling become a verb?'

"I've been a New Yorker all my life. Irish-Catholic, born in St. Claire's. I've never wanted to be anything but a nurse since the time I was three. I still have my little nurse medical bag and my nurse cap from when I was five to prove it. ER nursing intrigued me, but I didn't think I was the type for it. As it turned out, I was exactly the type.

"I've been twenty years in ER and there hasn't been one day that I've been able to imagine myself doing anything else. I like the patient population. I like that they come in in trouble, we figure out what's wrong, and then take an action to fix them. I'll admit too, that as an ER nurse, especially a New York City ER nurse, you get a pretty snotty attitude because what we do is life and death.

"Yeah, I come across as a hard-ass manager, but my bark is worse than my bite. When people make their way to my office, they pretty much leave with what they wanted. Ironically, I've been told that some of my staff are afraid of me. Then again, my supervisors no longer allow me to make schedule changes because I'm a weenie. My staff will say things like, "Oh dear, Suzanne, my shoelaces are untied. I think I need to go home." And I say, "Oh honey, that's terrible! Go ahead and take the day off."

New York City
September 11, 2001
8:50 a.m.

I was in the car listening to the radio, waiting to drive my mom to Penn Station. The broadcast was interrupted with a bulletin that a small plane had hit the World Trade Center. When my mother came out, I said, "Something just happened to the World Trade Center and I have to go into work."

I got out of the car and ran to the train station. You could see the smoke billowing out of the tower, but at that point I thought, *No big deal. We'll probably get some patients, but it won't be out of control.* Except everybody on the train was completely freaking out, so I found myself trying to calm people down by telling them it was going to be all right because it was only a small plane.

By the time I got to Times Square, eight minutes away, the trains downtown were already turned off. I found a policeman and told him I had to get to St. Vincent's, so he radioed for a unit to take me. I got into the squad car and about halfway down, around 20th Street, we heard that the second tower had been hit. The cops and I were literally dumbfounded. I started crying. I knew then that it wasn't an accident. For the rest of the ride we were silent as we listened to the constant signals from other cops who were witnessing what was happening.

I walked into St. Vincent's ER at 9:06 a.m. My head nurse met me at the door and said I was pale as a ghost. By the time I got back to my office to change shoes, I was hyperventilating. The head nurse told me that the disaster plan was already in place and that I needed to compose myself. She brought me a glass of water and two Motrin and I called my mother.

My mother was cool as a cucumber. She heard the panic in my voice and reminded me that I'd done this before in the 1993 bombing of the World Trade Center. She said, "Just get your act together and do what you need to do." It was like someone slapping me across the face because I hung up, put on my lab coat, popped my two Motrin, got my clipboard and went out.

I spoke to the administrator and director who had been on the curb right outside the ER talking when they heard a low-sounding buzz. When they looked up they actually saw the first plane hit the North Tower. Dr. Westfall, the ER Director, knew we were going to get a load of patients. In the 1993 bombing, we'd received one hundred eighty-three patients over the course of three days. Since that time, we've taken disaster drills very seriously. We'd had a drill just six weeks before, which I think was part of the reason the staff was so calm and focused.

9:15 a.m.

The outside MASH unit was set up. Stretchers, wheelchairs were ready, and personnel were all assigned to posts. The manpower pool had reported, and the walkie-talkies had all been distributed, which turned out great because our phones were down.

I went on autopilot, getting rid of the patients who were already there, and making sure each of the treatment areas had team leaders. I had off-duty nurses and retired ER nurses showing up at the door in scrubs and stethoscope saying "Just tell me what you want me to do."

9:30 a.m.

We had thirty-four nurses and fifty physicians, which was too many, so we put one nurse and one doctor at every bedside. And then, we waited. We wouldn't get our first wave of survivors until 10:30 a.m.

In hindsight, we knew that it had to be utter chaos down there, and there was no way they could have gotten people to us faster. Too, the office of Emergency Management Services was in the Trade Center and they'd been evacuated to the triage center, which was in the lobby of the North Tower. Subsequently most of them were killed.

Keep in mind that we were isolated in the ER. We had no information about what was going on. There's one TV in the paramedic office, but the reception was fuzzy because the antennae was on top of the World Trade Center. Phones were in and out because we were on the same phone-switching stations as the Trade Center. All of Manhattan was closed off at Fourteenth Street, so St. Vinnie's was in the frozen zone.

People ask me what was I thinking. To be honest, I wasn't thinking anything. I was numb. I was totally focused on putting my people in the places where they'd be most effective. Like Nancy Issing—I made her captain of our critical care area primarily because of her enormous experience as an ICU nurse and because she is very mature and calm. My strongest ER nurses, I put at the door to triage.

10:00 a.m.
Our satellite treatment and holding areas for the overflow were all ready and waiting. I remember looking around at my troops like the captain of a ship and feeling so proud of them. I wasn't frightened at all because I believed that we could handle anything. At the time I had no idea what the magnitude of the whole thing was going to be, but we were as ready as we were ever going to be.

We started hearing rumors from the people who had a clear view of downtown from the upper floors of the hospital that the first building had collapsed. I went outside, and sure enough, there was only one tower. My mind went on overwhelm. I realized then that we were going to get a whole lot more than a few smoke inhalation patients. I ran inside and called Central Supply for more trauma and burn packs.

The next rumors we heard were that Father Judge, New York Fire Department chaplain, had been killed and some of the cops and paramedics we know had been lost. Over the next half hour, Dr. Westfall and I told the staff the bad news. We assured them that we needed to stay ready for anything.

When we got the news that the Pentagon had been hit, everything in the department went dead silent. Then, all of a sudden, there was a change in the quality of the sirens that we'd been hearing for two hours. Now they were screaming up Seventh Avenue, and I remember thinking, *Oh my God, here it comes.*

And sure enough, it was just like on television—the doors flew open and the paramedics came in with six patients at a time. Those first patients were so desperately injured. I've never seen anything like it in my entire life. There was one man who came in soaked in jet fuel and for a minute I thought his pants legs were hanging off the side of the stretcher dragging on the ground, when in fact it was the skin from his legs. It was like strips of boiled chicken skin just hanging there.

The next patient had been in an elevator, and when the doors opened, a giant fireball engulfed him. He managed to get his arms over his face, but his chest and belly and arms were horribly burned.

We heard from the paramedics and cops that thousands of gallons of jet fuel just poured down the stairwells and elevators shafts, soaking everyone in its path. We got a total of sixteen burn patients, and transferred twelve to the burn centers. Out of those sixteen, a total of six survived.

All the patients came in covered with gray concrete dust, sort of like the volcanic ash in Pompeii. Their eyes were raw, and they were hacking from having breathed in all that stuff.

The traumatic injury patients quickly followed the burns. Our first was a man who was literally flattened. He'd obviously been blown up against something. His face was caved in, but they went ahead and cracked his chest anyway although he had no chest wall. There was nothing to lift up.

We didn't have a moment to think about anything other than what we were doing. Those first few hours reminded me so much of the opening scenes to *Saving Private Ryan* where it's just coming at you so fast. One part of my brain was thinking, *Hey, wait! Is that part of somebody's arm that got blown off?* In the time it took me to figure out what the hell it was, it was time to turn my attention to the next patient.

We got people coming in with their limbs twisted at bizarre angles and with dislocated ankles and knees and elbows. These were people who'd been running down the stairs and fell, or been stampeded, or who were crushed with the impact. One patient told me that with the concussion of the collapse, there was such a whoosh of hot air, it blew people right out of the building. We had people who were hit by debris and falling bodies. One man came in with a door hinge embedded in his back.

I thought a lot about my brother and cousins, who are all cops, but I didn't allow myself to dwell on it or I would have gone nuts.

Our medics had the worst time. One of them came in with a badly dislocated shoulder, and I asked him what the hell happened. He just looked at me and said, "Suzanne, people are falling from the sky. I'd follow them down with my eyes, and I knew they landed, but when I'd go look there would be nothing there because they all hit at such velocity they literally dispersed and disappeared under the debris. One of them glanced off my shoulder. She made a sound like a water balloon when she hit the pavement."

When the second tower went down, there was so much fire and smoke, that one paramedic said was just like in the movie *Independence Day*— it was coming at you and there was no place to escape. He said he was running alongside a van, and someone just reached out and pulled him inside the vehicle. Within seconds a cloud enveloped them and actually pushed the van along.

2 p.m.

It was like a faucet got turned off. We went from seeing about a hundred patients an hour, to maybe twenty or thirty. I couldn't fathom what had happened.

4 p.m.

Joe Davis, the Administrative Director and I took a walk and ended up on the roof of the Coleman building. We looked downtown and both silently cried. Even though we didn't say it, we each began realizing the enormity of what had happened.

Back in the department, Joe took one of our more seasoned medics aside and asked what was really going on. The man just looked at us and said with this very flat affect, "You aren't going to be getting anybody because there's nobody down there. It isn't what you think. It's flat—the whole thing went into the ground."

I didn't understand then. I was imagining forty story high mounds or something like what you see in earthquakes. I still wanted to believe people would survive.

Approximately 7 p.m.

We started getting people looking for their family members. We'd set up stations outside and had the patient lists from all the lower Manhattan hospitals. Remember that there were no Emergency Management Services at that point, so there was nothing else for the public—no numbers to call. They had nothing except to come to us and to the other hospitals in lower Manhattan.

We were still getting some patients, but they were primarily rescue workers with bad burns, lacerations, and lots of eye injuries. The dust had lime in it and was causing chemical burns to people's corneas, so we had six ophthalmologists down here just washing out eyes.

I don't see myself as a hero, but I do see my staff as heroes. They were amazing; especially in the way they protected each other. The one incident that clearly stands out in my mind was when the plastic surgeons were debriding the burn victims manually with their gloved hands and throwing the burnt flesh on the floor.

Nancy Issing had asked one of the housekeepers to clean it up and lied right to his face about what it was. She didn't think he could have psychologically handled what it really was, so she told him it was a new kind of protective dressing. Just that she took the time and thought to do that in the middle of everything was amazing to me.

A couple of our people went to Ground Zero that night. When they came back, they confirmed what the medic had told us—we weren't going to get any more survivors. And you know, I *still* didn't believe it.

Wednesday, September 12, 2001
2 a.m.

I went to bed in a room upstairs in Labor and Delivery. I turned on the TV and that was the first time I actually saw everything. It was surreal. We'd treated about four hundred and fifty patients that first day, but the TV was saying there were at least nine thousand dead.

5 a.m.

I went back to the ER still thinking that there were going to be lots of survivors coming in, so I was making sure the areas were staffed and ready.

The entire day went by and all we saw was a steady stream of rescue workers who just wanted to be treated and get back down to the site. Most of our service was to the families who came in looking for loved ones.

6 p.m.

I went down to Ground Zero with the administrator to deliver some eye drops to the treatment center. I saw a fire truck that had been smashed to pieces like a child's toy. You could tell the ladder had been up and torn away. It was Ladder 5, which was the ladder company of one of the fireman married to our administrator's secretary.

Seeing it firsthand, I realized that what people had been telling us was true—there wasn't even a boulder to pick up to see if anyone was under it. It was overwhelming. I don't have other words to explain it. You see pictures of wartime Europe, and it's never real—it's a photograph. Then you see firsthand how something manmade and mammoth can be utterly destroyed, and you suddenly know the reality.

By the time you reach my age, you've probably been in despair a number of times, but at that moment I truly had no hope. Oh, I'd heard about all the firefighters they were finding, but you know, they weren't finding bodies, they were finding their bunker gear which doesn't burn.

Thursday, September 13, 2001

We got a young guy who'd been urinating blood since Tuesday. It was his only symptom. From his CAT scan, we could see that he had a chunk of metal right in the middle of his kidney. The only mark he had was a tiny pinprick on his upper abdomen. The thing went through his small bowel, large bowel, skimmed across his spleen and landed inside his kidney.

6 p.m.
I went home for the first time since the towers were hit. My brother and mom were there. My brother couldn't even talk—he'd been down at Ground Zero putting body parts into bags, doing things that I doubt I'd be capable of doing.

Tuesday, September 18, 2001
Initially the smell of burnt chemicals and fuel was everywhere, but I was talking to my mother on the phone and she was complaining about a strange smell drifting across Brooklyn and into Western Queens. She said the workers were telling people that it was spoiling meat from the destroyed restaurants. At that point I said, "Come on, Mom, you *know* what that smell is."

February 2002
I haven't been back to Ground Zero. It's too hard. I'm so angry at what happened. I find myself getting really annoyed with tourists who travel from all over the US to see Ground Zero. They act really disappointed and say things like, "Gee, it just looks like a regular construction site."

Then the anthrax scare hammered us. We saw about a thousand people a week who believed that every pimple was anthrax-related. It was total hysteria. Take for instance, the guy who bit into his sandwich and called an ambulance because he thought the Parmesan cheese (which he actually *watched* them sprinkle on his sandwich) was anthrax powder.

The whole thing has definitely put all my ducks in a row. I can't be so worried about the future all the time. I mean, I'm not going to take all my money out of the bank or stop dieting (everything chocolate was going into my mouth during those first few weeks), but I've learned as an ER nurse that one tiny second can change life as you know it forever.

I just don't think I'll ever feel safe again, and I'll never take for granted that I'm waking up in the morning.

September 11, 2014

I've just read this interview that I gave thirteen years ago, and it gave me pause to realize how much has changed. St. Vincent's is gone. So is my mother. My brother and cousins have retired from the NYPD, but some of the staff from St. Vincent's Emergency Department work with me at the hospital where I am an emergency nurse and the Director of Emergency Services.

Osama Bin Laden is dead, but somehow, we are far from being safe. I still don't think that my actions that day or in the months to follow were particularly heroic, but I remain humbled by the actions of the ER staff.

There are so many things I remember about that day. I remember the cellist who walked from Lincoln Center and asked how he could help. He was shown to our chapel. Eventually many of his musician friends joined him, and for several weeks we had amazing music twenty-four hours a day.

I especially remember our Vice President of Mission, Sister Miriam Kevin Phillips, being interviewed by a national news reporter on the night of September 11. The reporter asked, "Aren't you disappointed that you didn't get more patients?"

In response, Sister Kevin swept her arm over the many hundreds of rescue workers, staff, family and friends crowding Seventh Avenue, all of them hoping to find out about loved ones. "Look around you," she said. "They are *all* our patients."

That one statement changed the way I viewed the role of emergency nurse and the many ways we care for our patients, their families and our community.

Over the past thirteen years, whenever I think of September 11, 2001, I'm thankful that on a day when I saw the worst of what people can do to each other, I was also able to witness the very best of what people have to give, and that is what I try to focus on.

FAYE

"Working in emergency room has changed me. I'm hardened because all I see is the worst of the worst. In the emergency room, we don't see the pregnant woman who comes in to say, "I had an amniocentesis today and everything was perfect," we see the woman on her eighth try at having a baby and she has just lost the fetus because she had the amniocentesis. So, when I had my amniocentesis, I was freaked out of my mind.

"I see motorcyclists come in either DOA or crushed, burned, or missing limbs. When my husband takes his bike out, I'm totally paranoid. I wait by the phone for 'the call' from the coroner. When my kid goes to a swimming party, I dwell on all the drowned kids or the kids with diving related spinal injuries that I've seen.

"Saving a patient keeps me high for weeks. A save makes me constantly aware that for every three people we lose, there is one person who will live because of us. That's what makes me think, 'Yeah, it's understaffed, and the politics are really ugly, but I can't wait to go to work today.'

"The story I'm about to tell you happened a week ago. It got my blood going to the point where I'll probably be okay to work here for another six months."

Young guy in his thirties. Vegetarian. Yoga instructor. Runs stress management workshops. Never sick a day in his life. Mr. Healthy. Mr. Laid Back. Mr. Sprouts. That is how this patient, whose stilled heart lies a few inches under my gloved hand, was presented to me seventy-four minutes ago.

Rather than keep my eyes glued to the monitor, as the others are wont to do—a straight line is surely not that interesting—I examine every inch of his face. Broad nose, almond shaped eyes with black pupils wide open and fixed. Despite the mottled, ashen hue, I can see that his underlying skin color falls between two races—brown and white. His skin is smooth to the touch despite the fact it is cold and clammy. When I lean in close, I can smell the incense still clinging to his hair.

I run the facts of his day through my mind, recreating the scenes with background orchestration: I envision him leaving the house dressed in the loose white sweats that now lay in the corner of my trauma room, torn to pieces, and soiled with blood, vomit, and urine.

I picture him teaching his yoga class, confidently showing his pupils a new, advanced pose. Then, I imagine him driving home, lightly rubbing the center of his chest, hoping to ease the mild ache that will not go away no matter how many arnica tablets his homeopath encourages him to take.

Two hours and a hot soak later, his wife, who is more in touch with the realities of everyday life than he, takes the reins and steers him down a more conventional path.

First stop: western emergency medicine, HMO style. No tests are ordered, not even an EKG, because in reality, those things cost time and money, and after all, he is *only* thirty years old.

With much rolling of eyes and reprimands about wasting the overburdened doctor's time, the couple is dismissed with the explanation, "You're too young and healthy to have a heart attack." They are given instructions to take antacids and stay away from spicy food.

An hour later, as her husband turns a darker shade of gray and his chest pain grows worse, his wife calls 911. Against his protests, Mr. Too Young and Healthy is loaded into the ambulance.

Still in the driveway, the paramedics administer one nitroglycerine, which renders him pain-free, pink, and feeling frisky. He tells a joke. He thanks the paramedics and says he'll just hop out right here and go have a tofu burger and sprouts with the wife.

The paramedics joke right back and tell him the only place he's hopping out is the ER. He pouts and complains, but okay—he'll make his contribution to the paramedics' annual beer bash fund and allow them to take him for a ride.

The ambulance reaches the end of his driveway, a distance of twenty feet, when the rhythm on the monitor turns into a flat line. The change comes on so fast, that the paramedic who is taking his blood pressure, passes it off as a loose lead and nothing more. Except Mr. Too Young and Healthy's blood pressure is zero over zero. When the paramedic looks up in surprise, his patient is no longer breathing.

Code three. Advanced cardiac life support measures are initiated. Mr. Too Young and Healthy does not respond to the paramedics' efforts. By the time he hits the double doors of our trauma room, he has been without a rhythm for eight minutes. I take one look at the blown pupils, the gray skin, and the fine ventricular fibrillation on the screen, and know that his chances of surviving are zero.

Trailing behind the rolling stretcher circus, his wife, her face set in a moue of determination, marches into the secret inner sanctum of the trauma room. She sits on the floor in the corner, daring us to deny her. "If he's going to die," she announces to the room, "he's going to die with me right here."

Inwardly I applaud her—it takes balls to go against a room full of adrenaline-charged medical warriors who are about to assault the man she loves.

Of course, because the wife is in the room, and because the patient is so young, all that can go wrong does.

First, we have an extremely difficult time intubating him, then the defibrillator malfunctions and we waste precious seconds waiting for the replacement. His intravenous line is accidentally pulled out before we have a chance to start a second line. Our ace IV nurse, who could start an IV on a combative elephant, has a hard time establishing a line. The external pacemaker is on loan to ICU, and the cardiac monitor brightness control is broken so that we all have to squint to see the rhythm—not that there is much of a rhythm to see.

The code goes on forever as Mr. Too Young and Healthy flips back and forth between a flat line and fine ventricular fibrillation. We've given him massive quantities of drugs and defibrillated him so many times, the smell of burned flesh permeates the room and sticks to the insides of our noses and clothes like lint.

I wonder whether we would still be working to save him if the wife wasn't in the room. I glance at her and notice that she's rocking and chanting. I can't hear what she's saying, but I assume it is some version of the usual, 'Please-save-him-make-him-live-don't-let-him-die' mantra all spouses chant at times like this.

With the Golden Hour long gone, I wonder if his brain is completely fried, or if our efforts at CPR have kept those cells oxygenated enough that, on the off chance he survived, he might still be able to remember his name and how to tie his shoes.

A sudden ripple of excitement runs through the room. His cardiac rhythm has changed from a flat line to coarse ventricular fibrillation, giving us a bit of an electrical edge to work with; a narrow ledge of hope from which to hang.

We shock and push more drugs again, and then again.

The doctor whoops. The cardiac monitor is showing a normal rhythm. An enthusiastic chorus of arm-pumping "Yes!" and, "All right!" fills the room then abruptly stops. Everyone goes silent.

The rhythm has no pulse marching along with it, which means the heart isn't beating. This sort of rhythm is called pulseless electrical activity. It's what I think of as a fake rhythm, an electrical sham from which few return.

We hold our breath and keep our fingers on his carotid artery. No pulse, no dice. Abruptly the rhythm flips again into coarse ventricular fibrillation and, because this is usually considered to be a deadly arrhythmia, it seems perverse that we consider it a lucky break.

I continue chest compressions, stopping only to let someone defibrillate. I can see by the doc's expression that she's ready to call off the code and let him go. We've gone beyond what is considered medically heroic and are now doing what could correctly be called beating a dead horse.

An idea rises from the darkest, deepest dead zone of my mind and flits around my head. It is an unorthodox notion, and I automatically dismiss it out of fear of embarrassing myself. At the same moment, I happen to look over at the wife and catch her staring directly at me. It's almost as if she has read my mind because her eyes plead with me to do something to save him.

"How about giving him a dose of B—?" The words are out before I realize I've said them aloud.

Two nurses screw up their faces at the very mention of this drug. The lab tech actually snorts. The pharmacist curls his lip and scoffs at the idea. "I doubt we even have it in stock," he says, as if I have just suggested injecting the patient with arsenic.

Someone else says, "It's not even legal anymore, is it?"

After a minute of thought, the doctor shrugs. "Why not? We have nothing to lose."

The pharmacist hurries off shaking his head in disgust, and the team stares at the doctor and me as if we are in cahoots on some bizarre practical joke.

An amp of the antiarrhythmic is found in a dusty box on pharmacy's odd stock shelf. Because no one else will, I inject the drug into Mr. Too Young and Healthy's IV and flush it through the tubing. All eyes on the monitor, we hold our collective breath.

Under my fingers, the first ripple of a pulse is so slight I think it must be a physical manifestation of my own hope. But then, the beat grows stronger until it is visibly bouncing my fingers off his carotid.

We smile and high-five in triumph when the doctor dampens our victorious spirits with the observation that Mr. Too Young and Healthy's pupils remain fixed and open—a sign that means we have just prolonged the life of a person without a functioning brain. The most we can hope for is that he will stay alive long enough in ICU to give the wife a chance to say her private good-byes.

For the rest of the shift, none of us can shake the gloomy sense of defeat that sits on our shoulders. We each try to block out Mr. Too Young and Healthy and his wife's hopeful face from our minds.

I go home and have a stiff drink and then another. At 4 a.m. my husband comes downstairs and sits across from me. He stares into my eyes for a long time without saying a word. I know enough to know he won't understand about Mr. Too Young and Healthy and how it feels to lose the battle. No one, except another of the inner circle of medical warriors would understand.

Finally my husband rises and heads for the stairs. "Maybe," he says over his shoulder, "You should think about looking for a different line of work."

The light of dawn is coming through the living room window when I finally fall asleep. I wake an hour later to go through the motions of my day. I comb my daughter's hair and wonder if Mr. Too Young and Healthy had a daughter, and when was the last time he combed her hair? I think about his wife, trying to imagine how she will cope with losing her husband so young.

My husband kisses me goodbye and I torture myself by imagining that he will end up in some ER that very day with another nurse leaning over him, wondering about his personal life.

By the time I walk into work, I feel a little insane. I play with the idea of walking straight to the Psych Department and committing myself. I wonder if they'd recognize a walking case of post-traumatic stress disorder when it came through their doors wearing scrubs.

I work like an automaton as I go from three glass-encrusted vehicular accident survivors, to a couple of abusive drunks, to a maggot-infested street person, to a drug overdose, to a gunshot wound, a stroke, an ultimately successful suicide attempt, and a screaming kidney stone. When my ten-minute break finally arrives, I run upstairs to the ICU.

The ICU charge nurse sits impassive while I bombard her with questions that must be answered before I can hope to sleep tonight. What time did Mr. Too Young and Healthy die? How did the wife take it? Did she get a chance to say goodbye? Was there family present to give her support?

When I've exhausted my list of inquiries, she asks what the hell I'm blathering on about.

"You know. The young guy who arrested yesterday? The brain dead guy we sent up to you? Mr. Yoga?"

She points over my shoulder. "You mean *that* Mr. Yoga?"

I turn around and blink. In bed twelve, Mr. Too Young and Healthy is sitting up eating lime Jell-O that his radiant wife spoons into his mouth.

I hurry to his bedside and touch his hand because I don't believe my own eyes. I say his name. He nods and says hello, not recognizing me. He is clearly puzzled by my expression.

The wife takes my hand then slips her arm around my shoulders. "Thank you," she says, really meaning it. "Thank you for bringing him back."

I return to the ER, all tiredness gone. And then those double doors swing open and on the stretcher I see a smooth brown face stained by a sea of blood. In the background I can hear a woman's pleading wail. "Please, please save him. Save my son."

I run toward the sound of suffering, praying that I can save him, save her—save them all.

MOLLY

"For me, nursing is like being in a bad marriage—I don't love the guy anymore, but I haven't met anyone worth leaving him for. He pays my bills, lets me come and go as I please, we still have some laughs and tender moments, but for the most part, he drives me nuts.

"After I'd already been working as a nurse for a few years and hating it, I went to a career counselor who gave me one of those career aptitude tests. Well, it came out that I was best suited for a career as a healthcare professional. I was furious, so I went back and verbally shredded the counselor.

"Finally, she very quietly said, 'Hey, it's who you are. Learn to accept it.'

"Right after that, I went to work in a small rural ER where I immediately learned that whether it's feast or famine, there's only one waitress. What I mean is, that either you fall asleep or you're up to your ears in alligators. ER nurses in rural areas are the whole show. I'm usually the only nurse on duty at night. There's no respiratory therapy, no lab, no x-ray. It's just me and the doc who is asleep down the hall.

"In the boonies you learn to be very resourceful. You have to fine-tune your skills, whether it's a sore throat or a gunshot wound. If I can't get that intravenous line in, well, nobody's going to do it for *me and the patient might die. It's a matter of life and death. Simple as that."*

MAY

First night in ER. Not bad, but then again, how bad can it get in a thirty-bed hospital? Gotta love that low volume of the sick and dying. After reading all the nursing horror stories, I reckon I must be working in the best hospital in the nation. The doctors and nurses get along well and mutually respect each other, we're overstaffed, our patients get the best care, including backrubs and whirlpools once a day whether they need it or not.

Tonight we had four patients. A six-month-old with an earache, Mrs. D. from the library with a laceration she sustained while washing her grandmother's crystal sherbet glasses, Frank J. with a fractured collarbone he got while breaking in one of his new horses, and Tom P. with congestive heart failure.

Tom was in bad shape. We loaded him up with Lasix and morphine until he had a reaction to the morphine. It was just like in the textbooks: that red streak going right up the path of his vein. Silly, but it was sort of a thrill to actually see it.

JUNE

What a night! I'm convinced now more than ever that nursing is a great way to learn about people and relationships—it's an insider's view. We're with people during the most profound moments of their lives; strangers, really, but you're there and it bonds you forever.

I delivered Kathy R's baby (a nine pound boy) on the gurney between the pickup truck and the ER doors.

Tom P. came in again by ambulance. He died in my arms about forty minutes later.

Mrs. K. came in short of breath. She finally consented to a chest x-ray after I spent an hour talking her into it. Dr. N. told her that she had some spots that looked like it might be cancer.

What got to me was that she was shocked. How could anybody who smokes three plus packs a day of unfiltered Camels for forty years be surprised? The only surprise is that she wasn't dead twenty years ago.

About half the patients I treated tonight came in as a result of drugs or alcohol-related accidents. God how I hate that crap—it ruins so many lives. Sometimes I have this fantasy, imagining what the world would be like without cigarettes, street drugs and alcohol.

I'm good when it comes to the dying folks. When I was holding Tom P., trying to make him feel comfortable, he grabbed my hand. He stared right into my eyes and said, "Molly, I want to take some of your goodness with me when I go."

And he did. He died looking into my eyes. I smiled for him the whole long moment so he could take that with him too.

One thing I've learned from working in the ER is that I will never leave someone I care about in anger or on bad terms. I tell people I love them more often. Life is delicate, precious, and way too short.

JULY

Goddamn it, I HATE shit. It is, by far, the biggest drawback in nursing! No matter what unit I work, there's always shit—excrement, poop, feces, crap. It's unavoidable.

Tonight I did a fecal disimpaction on Mrs. K. It was thoroughly disgusting. I filled, no lie, two bedpans, not to mention the stuff that fell onto my new shoes. Next time, I'm wearing shoe covers. NO MORE WHITE SHOES!

AUGUST

I can't sleep—can't stop thinking about Annie, the young girl who was raped. She's the pretty dark eyed girl who works at Dairy Queen on the weekends, the one whose window I always go to because I love her dimples. She's fifteen.

Some older boys were drinking out by the old quarry road, and spotted her walking. She was only a quarter mile from home. Ten minutes and she would have escaped the nightmare that will affect her every day for the rest of her life. She was so traumatized both physically and emotionally, that I didn't want to send her home. I was appalled that Dr. W discharged her without a second thought.

The father was a cold and nasty piece of work, accusing Annie of doing something to encourage the violence. Her mother was disgusted, holding everyone, including Annie, in contempt. They wavered between swearing vengeance on the boys and their families, and threatening to send Annie to a foster home in order to protect *their* reputation!

The whole thing made me want to cry. It was so out of the dark ages of parenting. The poor girl was shown no tenderness or understanding. I called Rape Crisis, but they wouldn't send anyone out because the parents refused to have anyone else involved, and the girl was too scared to demand her rights.

I've been crying since I got home. I can't stand this.

OCTOBER

I have decided that as a nurse, I'm also an artist. It's an art to be with someone while they're sitting on the toilet taking a dump. It's an art to conduct a chatty and enlightening conversation while you're inserting a catheter into a patient's penis. There is an art to providing a safe and caring atmosphere for a young woman or a child who has just been raped or beaten or both. It's an art not to flinch when collecting foul specimens from the suffering. It's an art not to cry when a patient you've grown close to, dies in your arms. It's an art that makes us able to easily handle what could be construed by most people as life's most embarrassing moments.

The art of nursing is not easy.

I went by Dairy Queen after work to get one of those chocolate-coated cones. The new counter girl told me Annie's parents made her quit.

NOVEMBER

Another dent in my heart. Tonight they brought us a twenty-two-year-old from a high-speed rollover vehicular accident out on Highway 12.

The young man got off easy with a scalp laceration and a lung contusion, but his twenty-one-year-old wife died at the scene. They were on their way to Fargo where the wife was to be matron of honor in her best friend's wedding.

We all knew she was dead, but we weren't allowed to tell the husband until he'd been cleared of any spinal cord injury—standard procedure in case he went crazy and try to bolt.

For the two hours he was immobilized on the backboard waiting for an x-ray, he begged every person who walked by to tell him how his wife was doing. Each in turn, we lied, saying we hadn't heard anything about her. I know he saw right through the bullshit. Finally, he grabbed Dr. W and asked him.

Dr. W. put his hand on the boy's shoulder and said, "Son, your wife was killed instantly. They've taken her to the morgue."

The guy began to sob. He told us that they had a two-year-old son. He wanted to know what he should tell his son when he asked where mommy was. And, how would he be able to face her parents?

When he didn't get any answers, he started chanting, "This is a dream, this is only a dream, this is only a dream." Then he'd look at me and ask, "Isn't it?"

I broke down. Couldn't help it. The bereavement counselor and the priest were there telling him all this crap about how his wife was with God in a better place and how lucky he was to be alive so he could raise his son. I wanted to tell them to shut the fuck up. I don't know, though, maybe people need to hear that bullshit.

Things like this have changed me. A person can be driving down the street, not a care in the world, and in a millisecond, your life is changed forever. One minute you're fine, the next you're a paraplegic or cognitively delayed or blind forever. It has made me think about the consequences of everything I do.

DECEMBER

Worst night of my life. I was so stressed that I just had to stand back and take deep breaths until I stopped shaking. I can't even cry anymore, I'm so drained.

Annie, the Dairy Queen girl who was raped, came in DOA. I cleaned her up. That sweet, delicate face was so twisted, it was like she wasn't even the same person. Hanging does that to a body.

The paramedic brought in the note. I shouldn't have read it, but I did. It was full of self-recrimination. Why the hell didn't somebody see what was going on? A friend? A teacher?

The parents came in asking, "How could she do this to us?"

I lost it and pointed out, at the top of my lungs, that Annie was the one who suffered, not them. Selfish assholes.

Dr. W ordered me out of the department and told me to cool down. I ran two miles in the snow before I could get the anger and despair out of my system.

When I stop and think about it, I realize I'm not really in any position to judge the parents. I could have called that girl and talked to her. I could have told her she could come to my house and talk any time she needed to. I don't know, would she have done that?

Mostly, what I really want to know is: was there a chance I could have saved her?

ANN CARROLL
Ground Zero
Labor and Delivery, ICU, ER, Flight Transport nurse

"I was a third-year pre-med student when I had to have surgery. That changed my view of doctors and nurses forever. The doctors were too detached. I am not a detached person, so I challenged the Regents program and became a nurse.

"I love nursing even though the docs have all the power—unfortunately, much of it misplaced. If I had the power, I'd make it mandatory that doctors would have to work as nurses for five years before they could practice as physicians.

"I work for an air ambulance company in California and a second job in community hospitals in ER, ICU and Labor & Delivery. I'm the type of nurse who gives the patients my home phone number. Part of that might come from growing up with so many brothers and sisters to care for. That's why I decided to quit med school and become a nurse instead—it's the compassion thing. It's what nurses do."

September 11, 2001
Somewhere over Las Vegas, Nevada

I was in the back of a medical transport Cessna 421 with a woman who was pregnant with twins, and whose membranes had ruptured prematurely, when the pilot suddenly turned to look in the back of the aircraft and shouted, "We've been bombed!"

It was the first time I'd flown with this pilot, so I said to my medic, "Oh Lord, I think our pilot might be smoking crack. Who would be crazy enough to bomb the United States?"

The pilot saw the look on my face and said, "Listen, I'm serious. The Pentagon has been hit and NYC has been bombed. I've been ordered to land immediately."

My medic and I were both thinking, *What the hell is wrong with this guy? Is he in need of a psych unit? Are we gonna make it down okay?*

I heard him making emergency plans to land in Las Vegas, and that was when I realized he was dead serious.

After transporting the patient to the nearest facility, I found a TV in a packed, but very silent, physician's lounge. When I saw with my own two eyes what had happened, I immediately made up my mind that I had to go to New York and help in any way I could.

My two-week vacation began September 12, so I looked at my medic and said, "There goes my vacation. I've got to get to New York."

I called the American Red Cross and they told me to bring my trauma papers and get there as fast as I could. It took some doing, but I managed to get on a commercial flight to New York on September 13. All during the flight I reviewed my trauma books, thinking in terms of what the survivors would need in the way of trauma care.

I held that thought right up until we flew over New York City and I saw the devastation from the air. I freaked out and just put away my books, knowing without any doubt that there was no way anyone could have survived that amount of destruction.

I got off the plane and spent my first day in New York with a group of nurses at the Javits Center, organizing supplies. After we'd organized everything, the military came in and said they were taking over.

Our group of civilian nurses really didn't like that idea, so we went to the State Police who told us the Red Cross needed nurses. The cops escorted us down to PS 234 at Chambers and Greenwich where the Red Cross Station was set up. They were sending teams of nurses down to Ground Zero for eight-hour shifts, which in hindsight was way too long.

The Red Cross was grateful for us because unbeknownst to anyone at the time, the military had been turning away all the fully qualified trauma nurses who volunteered to help. Don't ask me why. Also, there was a shortage of everything—nurses, masks and other supplies. That really pissed me off, because after a while, we weren't getting relieved. We were choking on the smoke and debris that was in the air, and we were exhausted.

That first night, I noticed right away that many of the rescue workers were exhausted as well. They had cuts and burns and their eyes were filled with ash. There was a serious shortage of masks, and the ones they did have weren't the right kind. We ended up working all night, just getting everybody masks and fed.

I had a room, but it was expensive and a long way from the site. I knew my money wasn't going to last if I stayed there, so after two days of getting three hours sleep and then trying to get back to the site, one of the nurses said I should just stay at PS 234 and sleep in the gymnasium.

I'd buddied up with Angel Lopez, a Hospice nurse from Arizona who'd been on vacation up in Canada, so for the first two nights at PS 234, we slept on the floor of the gym and I ended up with a case of athlete's foot on the side of my chest. After that, we mostly all had cots to sleep on, but it was stifling in there because all the windows and exits had been taped off with plastic to keep the ash out.

And cockroaches? Holy crap, I didn't know they could get that big! I remember Angel telling me one morning that I needed to take a shower or she was going to move my cot to the other side of the gym. So, I took a shower and found out there was no hot water. I came out of the shower blue and shaking, and told Angel, "I just took a shower with the biggest cockroach in New York City. I think he asked me out on a date."

Each day I made my rounds of the rescue workers, bandaging blisters, treating cuts and burns—some of them full thickness—and washing out the workers' eyes. The bottoms of the workers shoes, and subsequently their feet, were wrecked, either cut up or burned away, from walking over the rubble. I don't know how in the world they were standing up on those burns and blisters, but they wouldn't quit. They'd go right back out there after we'd bandaged them. We didn't have much to bandage them with at that point, and there were no masks, so we were making do with what we had.

About day five, the lack of supplies and masks was really becoming an issue. I was so angry about the situation, that I walked over to the news trucks where Bill Hemmer from CNN was standing, went right up to him and said, "You should help us get us some supplies. We don't have anything to take care of these blisters on the rescue workers' feet."

Before I knew it, they were sticking microphones up under my blouse and Hemmer told me that if I wanted the supplies, I'd have to go on the air and ask for them. So they put me in front of a camera and I gave a list of what we needed.

Within four hours we got all the supplies I'd asked for in huge quantities—hundreds of boxes of foot dressings and shoe pads, masks, Duoderm for blisters, eye wash, you name it—all of it delivered to our door.

At night, before the Red Cross trucks got there, Angel and I made rounds with Gatorade and water and food. The workers were suffering from heat exhaustion and dehydration because they weren't drinking enough fluids, so we'd make them drink, and then I'd wash out their eyes. Anybody and everybody who worked down there had eye problems.

Also, the workers were internalizing everything, and as a result, they'd developed gastrointestinal troubles from the stress.

After a couple of days I was asked to go out onto the rubble, so I put on my mask and hardhat and when I got there, I was in a state of shock. Walking on top of it all was overwhelming. It didn't seem real. I wanted to cry, but I couldn't let myself do that, so I fought the urge by forcing myself to keep moving. Moving. Constantly moving.

The first week, everyone believed there were people still alive in there, and when it came clear that there wasn't, well, that was demoralizing as hell.

Angel tired much more easily than I, so she rested a lot more. I couldn't sleep at all. As soon as that gymnasium door opened and someone yelled, "We need a nurse out here," I'd be off that cot and upstairs in a flash. It was actually a great system.

About the eleventh day I was there, things slowed down because the rescue workers were more cautious and the urgency to save survivors was gone. They were just finding body parts at that point. This was when the real depression began to set in.

I actually lost seventeen pounds from the smell. It was so terrible, it hurt my stomach. I would try and eat soup, especially Campbell's Wedding Soup and it would come right back up. To this day I cannot eat that soup. It also took years before I could handle the smell of Chicken McNuggets, which were also offered to rescue workers. Robert De Niro donated food from his restaurant in Tribeca. I'd always liked him as an actor, but I loved him for making the donations.

One night Angel and I—still dressed in our scrubs—went to dinner at a really nice, upscale restaurant in Tribeca. We had a great meal, but when I asked the waiter for the check, he told us that I would incite a riot if I tried to pay the bill. Everyone in that restaurant wanted to pay for our meal! I will always love New Yorkers.

Vick's VapoRub became more guarded than the narcotics. Angel and I smeared it inside our mask filters to cover up that smell. I don't know how it works on colds, but Vick's VapoRub definitely saved the day on that one.

As I've said, the masks were always a problem. Angel and I actually went down to the FEMA station where they had the canister filters, but no masks. The Red Cross station had the masks, but no canisters. So, we did a little sharing. A lot of the men didn't want to wear the masks because they were uncomfortable, claustrophobic, and, because they couldn't smoke.

I'd tell them, "Put your masks on! You're hurting your lungs breathing all this ash."

And they'd say, "Well, it's really not *that* bad." So I finally started reminding them that part of that ash that they were breathing in, was actually people's bodies that had vaporized. Believe me, *that* got the masks on their faces real fast!

I walked up to Mayor Giuliani and Police Commissioner Kerik and offered them masks. I explained that they should be wearing them, and Mr. Kerik asked who I was. I told him I was an ICU nurse from California, and if he didn't wear the mask, then I would move to New York City and take care of him when he became sick from not wearing one.

Mayor Giuliani looked from me to Mr. Kerik and said, "Put on the mask." The police officers who were watching the whole scene told me I had balls. I didn't see it that way. I saw it more as I was just doing my job.

For six weeks afterward, I coughed up black stuff. In California, I used to run about six and a half miles three times a week. When I got back home, I tried to run, got two miles into it, and had an asthma attack. I've never had asthma in my life. My voice will never be the same again. So now I'm thinking that all those heavy metals everyone breathed for all those weeks, are going to kill us, mask or no mask.

You'd tell the rescue and cleanup guys whatever you had to in order to get them to take care of themselves. Some of their lacerations were pretty severe, but they absolutely refused to sit long enough to be sutured. One of the workers came to us with a really bad laceration on his foot, so he definitely needed a tetanus shot. I mean, think about all the sewage down there—one hundred ten stories of it!

The guy said he didn't have time for a shot and he didn't need it anyway. I thought about that for a minute, then very calmly and professionally, I said, "Well, okay, you can probably get by without a tetanus, but three days from now when your penis starts swelling and turning black, you should get to the hospital as soon as possible and try to save it before it has to be surgically removed."

This guy almost fell on his knees begging for a tetanus shot.

Two days later, I had to pick up supplies from another treatment center and the doc working there asked me what kind of injuries I was seeing in the rubble. I told him about the lacerations and puncture wounds and what a hard time I was having getting the guys to take tetanus shots. I told him that I'd started telling them their penises were going to fall off.

The doctor started laughing and said, "Oh my God, that was *you*? We've had about fifty guys come through here in the last two days demanding tetanus shots."

To be honest, I never thought I'd get out of there alive. It was a dangerous situation. We were walking in the dark over those cables and wires. Some of those buildings were so unstable, and with all that big equipment swinging around in that rubble? One of them actually hit me in the butt one night.

I needed an extra pack to carry the supplies in and out of the pile, so I scrounged around PS 234 and found a boy's Superman backpack in the principal's office. I used that backpack the whole time I was there. When I left, I wrote a letter to the pack's owner, which, according to the name on the inside, was Nicholas. I told him how important his backpack had been and that it had helped a lot of rescue workers. I added that I was hoping it would get him out of any trouble he was in with the principal. I put the note in the backpack and returned it to the principal's office.

That same night that I went through the school looking for a backpack, I walked into a first or second grade classroom. On the blackboard, written in block letters I found:

TODAY IS TUESDAY, SEPTEMBER 11, 2001
WE WILL GO TO RECESS AFTER WE

The teacher was probably writing that when the first plane hit. What really got to me was that these kids had a perfect view of the World Trade Towers. One of the teachers who came down to check on things in the school said that the children thought the people jumping out of the buildings were birds that were on fire. What an image.

Another memory was the five physicians who came in to relieve the nurses for the night. When we returned the next morning, one of the Red Cross workers came up to me shaking her head and said, "Cripe, five doctors and they couldn't figure out what to do. The nurses had to tell them."

I had my bitchy days too. I remember the day Miss USA came down to the site to meet us. I'd just seen them pull half a body out of the rubble and I was a mess—drained, exhausted, hair sticking up, no make-up, and covered with soot. And here's this woman with perfect hair and make up, dressed in some sweet fashion statement, singing *God Bless America*? Oh puleeezzzz. What planet was *she* from? To top it all off, she came over and hugged me. All I could do was tell her it was a nice song.

The same day Miss USA was there, Angel and I had our photos taken with Nathan Lane, one of my favorite actors. I remember he was teary.

Out of all the things I saw during those weeks, the images that got to me the most—the pictures I will carry in my head for the rest of my life, were the faces of the wives, husbands and children of the firemen who—(long pause).

I thought I had to be tough, but I am not a tough person. I'm a loving, caring person, so at the memorial for the firemen and policemen, I lost it. A pregnant widow of a fireman came up to me and grabbed my arm and tried to tell me how grateful she was to us for being there. That just devastated me—it sobered my whole life. There was so much grief.

Another thing I won't forget is that we had no way to wash our clothes while we were down there, so we threw them away. I remember telling the other nurses that as a California woman, I took my Victoria's Secret undies very seriously and would not throw them away no matter how dirty they got.

Well, about a month after I got back to California, the New York City nurses sent me a hundred-dollar gift certificate from Victoria's Secret. The card read:

'Dear Ann,

How can we New Yorkers thank you for all the hard work? It takes a very special person to be as caring and giving as you are. Meeting you has enhanced our lives. Please accept this small token of our appreciation. Get some new underwear—we're sure Victoria's Secret never expected to be worn at Ground Zero.'

When I look back at those three weeks, I realize that the whole country had come together with the hopes of making a difference. In the end, the difference they made was mostly to each other.

Would I do it over again? In a heartbeat. Yes, it aged me, but I'm glad I was there. I was privileged to be there. I don't think it messed up all of our lives, but it definitely affected all of our lives. Helping people is the most important thing in life, and I made a difference in those people's lives.

KIT

"My mother always told me, 'If you become a nurse, you will never be refused a loan on a house and you will always be beneficial to your husband.'

"I never gave it a lot of thought—I just always accepted I'd be a nurse. When I graduated from nursing school in 1974, I did the loop—med-surge to ICU then straight to one of the roughest, busiest ERs in the United States.

"People don't realize there are no boundaries for ER nurses. We're trauma whores—we can't say no to chaos and disaster. There is no point that can be called our limit. We have to take all comers. There's no such thing as saying, "Sorry, you can't come here."

"On the other hand, ICU nurses can, and frequently do, turn patients away by saying, 'Sorry we have three nurses who all have three patients each, so we're full.' The ICU nurse's focus is completely different. They're more technical and interested in all the systems. The ER nurse focuses in on one part—where the injury is. That's it.

"I don't get as paranoid about stuff as I used to. Working ER has made me a little more carefree because I know that in the next hour I could very well be dead.

"The biggest bummer for me is the people I work with. There isn't much teamwork but a lot of writing each other up. If you can believe this, I've even been written up for laughing.

"The doctors in our ER mostly order tests, they don't often touch the patients. Rarely do they talk to the patients or the nurses. There's this one doctor who, when I walk in and see him, my whole being sags. He's not a team player and he's abusive to the nurses. He's the type who bellows instead of just asking a nurse for whatever it is he needs. It's as if he's never been in any social situations where he's had to behave like a normal human being. The nurses describe him as three toy poodles barking their heads off while running around on a linoleum floor. That's his personality in a nutshell—drives me absolutely batshit crazy.

"We have another doctor who's so germ-phobic that he won't shake anyone's hand. When his patients sign his discharge orders, he throws that pen right into the garbage. Where the hell is that at?

"The patient population is changing too. I see more and more thirty and forty-year-olds coming in with chest pain and other major cardiac problems. That translates into a lot of angry and stressed out people. Plus, does anybody realize how many teenagers are on anti-psychotic drugs these days? It's freaky scary.

"When I come home I can't really debrief with my husband because he's a paramedic and doesn't want to hear about it, so I usually call my coworkers or work it out myself.

"It's always in the back of my mind how easy it would be for some disgruntled patient to walk into the ER and blow us all away because he didn't get his drugs or he had to wait too long to be seen. I hate that paranoia—it's like an ER hangover that invades my life. When I'm out for a walk, I don't let my daughter wander two inches away from my side because I know what kinds of crazies are out there.

"I'm an Irish Bostonian who was raised Catholic, but I have to tell you that sometimes when I see the things that happen to people, I have to wonder if there really is somebody up there running this circus. And if there is, what kind of jerk allows this shit to happen?

"Just to remain sane, I have to make sense out of some of the bad stuff I see, but it gets harder and harder to do as time goes on."

It was my first day in the emergency department of a major inner city hospital that is nationally famous for the wild and crazy things that happened there. This place was so rough, two city cops have to be on duty twenty-four hours a day.

As the doors swung open to admit me to the Insanity Fun House, (keep in mind that this is in the first sixty seconds of my first day on the job) a patient comes charging at me with a steel gurney strapped to his back. I was paralyzed by the sight. My mind scrambled, trying to come up with an explanation—like, maybe something I'd had for breakfast had been spiked with LSD.

A petite woman, no more than five-feet-one and weighing about ninety pounds, materialized out of nowhere. The sleeves of her scrubs were rolled up with a pack of Virginia Slims tucked into the fold. She walked right past the guy with the gurney, held out a hand and smiled. "I'm Dr. M. Are you the new ER nurse?"

I shook her hand and nodded, still staring at the man wearing the gurney backpack. He'd smashed into the wall in his attempts to get out the door and knocked himself crooked, so that he was leaning, gurney first, against the wall—like an overturned turtle.

She looked at the guy then back at me. "What's wrong?" she asked, as if she really didn't know.

I pointed at the patient. "We need to do something. He's going to kill himself from the exertion."

"Pffft," she said, taking me by the arm. "Jack's tough as rhino hide. His only problem is that his PCP levels are up. He's busy trying out for the Olympic crucifixion event until someone from psych services gets here."

She brought her face close to mine and laughed. "Shit, I've never seen pupils so fully dilated on anyone standing upright. Do you feel okay, or are your vitamins just kicking in?"

I stared at the PCP gurney guy, then back at the doctor. The thought crossed my mind that maybe the entire psych unit had escaped and I was going to find the regular ER staff in a back room tied and gagged. The headlines ran through my mind:

'PSYCH PATIENTS HOLD ER STAFF HOSTAGE
ADMINISTRATION REFUSES NEGOTIATIONS'

We walked past the gurney guy and into the main room where the doc introduced me to the other staff. "The only things you need to be careful of are the new interns," Dr. M. warned. "They're tricky. They have very little knowledge and lots of authority, so as a nurse you have to make sure they don't kill people. They think they can do anything they want and have absolutely no fear of the consequences of their actions. They're like a bunch of three-year-olds playing with loaded automatic rifles."

She handed me a chart and patted me on the back. "Here's your first patient. Just remember, mistakes that hurt people are very hard to live with. Try not to kill anyone."

I laughed. She didn't.

My first patient was a merchant seaman who was having lower abdominal pain. When I handed him a gown and told him to undress, he outright refused.

"But you need to be undressed before the doctor will see you."

He shook his head. "I can't do that ma'am. You'll take offense at my tattoo."

I held up my hand. "Listen, it'll take a lot more than a tattoo to offend me."

It took five more minutes of cajoling, but I finally talked him into getting undressed. He pulled his pants down a little, and there, tattooed right above the pubis was:

BEWARE OF SWINGING BOOM

I was the very picture of professionalism while I took his vital signs. Then, I went out into the hall, buried my face in a towel and howled.

Of course, being new and wanting to impress the other nurses, I had to have a few of them come in and take a peek. Who would have something like this tattooed on himself unless he wanted someone to look, right?

The other nurses came in and were making a fuss over it when the patient said, "Ah hell, I might as well show you ladies the rest of it."

He pulled his pants the rest of the way off, and on the head of his penis was tattooed a dollar sign. Nobody said anything while we tried to figure out the hidden meaning.

"Oh come on ladies," he said finally, "You know how women love to blow money, don't you?"

My second patient was a very attractive blonde woman who came in with a Dragon Lady fake nail stuck in her nasal passage. For the entire time I was taking her vital signs, she desperately tried to convince me she wasn't picking her nose. As if I was born yesterday.

She swore she was smelling her nails and got rear-ended.

Right. Smelling her nails. Next patient, please.

I was getting ready to go to lunch when my first serious trauma patient came in. The woman was, thank God, only semi-conscious. The paramedics told us that the patient's husband was backing up the car, and somehow knocked her through the plate glass picture window at the front of their house.

At that point she wasn't too badly hurt, but when she tried to pull herself up, the upper half of the window fell and amputated both legs mid-thigh.

We'd stabilized her and had just sent her to microsurgery when two cops came running in, each holding a side of a floral print bed sheet. I peered at the contents, knowing I shouldn't. The legs were loosely wrapped in bath towels, bags of ice packed around them. That wasn't so bad—I'd seen amputated parts before. It was the shoes still on the feet that got me feeling so queasy that lunch was no longer an option.

Since I wasn't going to be eating, I thought I'd get some fresh air and wandered out to the entrance to join the small group of ER personnel who'd gathered for smokes. As we were chewing the fat, a beat-up purple Oldsmobile going about sixty flew up the drive and squealed to a halt some fifteen feet away.

Dr. M stubbed out her cigarette and said, "A dollar says it's an OD."

One of the orderlies shook his head. "Nope, my dollar says a shooting."

They both looked at me.

"Stabbing," I said, without thinking. Nobody could say I wasn't quick to catch on.

The back passenger door opened, a young man was pushed out onto the blacktop, and the car sped away. One of the city cops ran out to get the license plate number, but the car was already out of sight.

Dr. M hailed a gurney and did a quick assessment of the man's airway and circulatory status then looked at me smiling. "Multiple stab wounds. Very astute, girlfriend. You've just won yourself two bucks. Now help me get this kid on the gurney before he bleeds to death."

The whole time we worked on the kid, Dr. M gave what I would soon come to recognize as her 'treadmill speech.'

"We get these people dumped at our door," she said. "Then we fix them up using thousands of taxpayer's dollars, only to dump them back out on the streets so they can shoot or stab someone else who will be dumped at our door and the scenario plays all over again. It's one royally fucked up system."

By the time I retuned from turfing the stabbed kid to surgery, I found everybody in the main trauma room working on a two-year-old girl who'd been shot through the head by her father as an act of revenge against the mother.

I was told to get another IV line into her any way I could. I crouched down at the side of the gurney and desperately searched for a vein. Her little face was right in front of me, so I couldn't help looking at her. Big mistake, especially with a pediatric trauma—you don't ever look at them too closely or you lose all objectivity.

But I did look and she was so cute with her tiny earrings and her girly pink dress. I could tell that someone had really loved that baby. I could not comprehend how anyone could do that to an innocent child. I could understand wanting to kill yourself or another adult, but to kill a child?

I managed to get a line in, but there was so much yelling and insanity in the trauma room, it unnerved me until I wasn't able to think. I must have looked like I was in a daze, because Dr. M sent me out of the trauma room and ordered me to take care of the half-dozen crazies waiting to be seen.

To be honest, I don't do well with psych patients. They aren't a quick fix. You can't give them something and send them home. Depression is a terrible disease. You can't say, "Well in six months you'll be all better." They come in and they're so pathetic, you want to fix them, but you can't.

I walked into the pelvic room where Crazy Number One was waiting, opened my mouth to introduce myself, and recoiled at the stench assaulting my olfactory glands.

Excusing myself, I went to the supply cart and found a small packet of Vick's VapoRub, rubbed some under and inside my nose, and went back to the exam room.

I checked the young woman's vital signs, aware of the exaggerated bulge under the woman's thin sarong. Through the material I made out the words, 'Happy Birthday!' printed on the pink balloon that had been stuck under her clothes. Her blood pressure was low, her pulse fast, and her temperature was one hundred and three.

"It says here that you think you're in labor?"

The woman nodded. "The pains are coming pretty regular."

"How many weeks along are you?"

"Two."

I nodded, and, maintaining my poker face, asked her to put her feet in the stirrups and lay back. I rested my hand on the balloon. "I need your permission to touch your belly and do a quick pelvic exam," I said in my kindest, first-grade-teacher tone. With crazies it was always advisable to be careful. A litigious crazy could end a medical career with one accusation and the backing of any number of fanatical right-wing civil rights groups.

"Okay, but be very careful of the baby."

I rested my hand gently on the balloon. "I see that there's a helium balloon tied to your waist. May I untie it?"

The woman nodded, and I cut the ribbon holding the balloon, letting it float to the ceiling. Without any further discussion, I placed a paper drape over her abdomen and legs and brought the exam lamp close, immediately wishing I hadn't.

Clearly infected, the bulging, purple labia had been sewn closed with black nylon thread. Something that looked vaguely familiar protruded from between two of the lower stitches, but my mind refused to go there.

I turned off the lamp and smoothed down the drape. "It looks like your vagina has been sewn together and it appears to be infected. Can you tell me what happened?"

Wide-eyed, the patient twisted a strand of hair. "Well, I read this book that had pictures of women having babies and I wanted to know how it felt."

I nodded encouragingly though I prayed she would not go on. I really didn't want to hear the details, but I had to chart *something*.

"I stole a game hen from my mom's refrigerator and put it inside there and sewed it closed so it couldn't come out before it was due."

To look at me one might not have guessed I was screaming every bit as hard as Janet Leigh in the shower scene of *Psycho*, but I was. I blinked a few times, giving myself time to regain my inner cool. "Was it a few chicken parts or was it the whole bird?"

Oh my god, I thought, *did I really just ask that?*

Her eyebrows knit in a frown. "Whole. Why would I want only part of a baby to come out?"

I apologized for my breakdown in logic and assured her Dr. M would come in to see her as soon as she could.

I found Dr. M in the back room. "You need to see the patient in the pelvic exam room right away," I said, handing her the chart. "She's pretty sick, and she's going to need a psych consult as well."

Dr. M read my notes and looked up in disbelief. "She's about to deliver a slowly cooked hen?"

"Full fryer gestation," I said. "I saw the drumstick with my own eyes. It looked like it was done."

After I started IV antibiotics on our insane game hen lady and turfed her to surgery, I picked up my next chart. The intake clerk told me that the patient, known only as Velveeta, was one of the local prostitutes who came in regularly for minor gynecological ailments. The woman's main complaint this time was cramping, a persistent vaginal discharge, and withdrawal.

The clerk was puzzled by the last complaint because as far as she knew, Velveeta had never been into drugs, and, in fact, had a reputation among the other prostitutes as a crusader against drugs.

Velveeta was a big woman with hair the same color as the cheese. She wasn't obese, but muscular, like a woman mud wrestler.

"Hey, Velveeta, what's happening?"

"I got me some cramps with discharge," Velveeta explained in a smooth, low voice. "I need to do a withdrawal too, 'cause I'm taking me a vacation trip to Mexico and my man say I can't go if I'm all fucked up."

I mulled that over while I took her vital signs, trying to figure out what the hell cramps, being in withdrawal and a trip to Mexico had in common.

I asked the usual list of questions—when was her last menstrual period, what form of birth control did she use, when did the cramps start, and what drugs was she taking.

"I been taking aspirin for my fever," she said, "And, I been taking the magic juice every day."

I knew most of the names for the various street drugs, but magic juice was new to me. Velveeta certainly didn't appear to be under the influence of drugs, plus there were no track marks on her anywhere that I could see. It was a stretch, but all I could think of was that she was doing some street combo of heroine and cocaine that one drank, sniffed, smoked or rubbed into the gums or somewhere.

"Are you withdrawing from the magic juice?"

Velveeta looked at me strangely. "You crazy girl? Why I wanna do that? That shit cost me about two hundred dollars a pint."

I wondered what kind of street drug came in pints and was about to ask her what was in this magic juice when Dr. M came in looking a little spiky. The wisenheimer smirk was gone from her face, so I figured she was still flipped out over the Human Crockpot hen lady.

The doc hastily introduced herself and looked to me for the lowdown and the GYN exam packet.

"Velveeta's been having cramps in her lower abdomen and persistent vaginal discharge for about two weeks," I said, laying out the speculum and the sterile gloves. "She also wants to be checked for withdrawal."

I knew from Dr. M's vague gaze, and the way she kept mumbling, "Hmmm" and, "Oh that's nice" as docs are wont to do when they aren't really listening, that she hadn't taken in a word I'd said.

Speculum inserted, Dr. M had Velveeta only partially dilated when the first hundred-dollar bill fell out.

God only knows how long Velveeta had been banking at Vaginal First National, because she must have had at least three thousand dollars in that vault. Dr. M pulled out wads of hundred dollar bills until there was nothing left in the vaginal vault except the appropriate organ.

After taking a culture and slide of the discharge, Dr. M excused herself. The door hadn't closed all the way before Velveeta jumped off the table and started counting the bills, throwing them in the exam room sink for laundering. She was draping the money over the rails of the gurney to dry when Dr. M came back in with a prescription for antibiotics.

Velveeta turned narrowed and accusing eyes on her. "What'd you do with the rest of my money, bitch?"

Dr. M didn't miss a beat. "I made a withdrawal and closed the account, just like you asked."

"This here is only three thousand five hundred dollars. I put four thousand in there. What you do with them other five bills?"

"Since I doubt that was an interest-bearing account, maybe your johns got more than they bargained for," Dr. M suggested.

Velveeta shook her head. "Don't you get smart with me, girl. If you don't give me them bills, I'll set the police on you."

Dr. M leaned against the wall looking pensive. "Well," she said, "I don't have them, but I think I know where they are."

Velveeta ceased shuffling the dripping currency and gave Dr. M her full attention.

"It's a very rare medical condition," Dr. M continued. "Have you ever heard of circulating bills?"

"Sure," Velveeta said with the defiant attitude of one who knew no such thing. "I know all 'bout them."

"Well, that's where I think those extra bills went—into your circulation."

Dr. M shot me a look. I was sucking in my lips, biting back the howling laugher that was clawing to get out.

Dr. M handed her the prescription slip. "Take these for the full two weeks."

"This medicine gonna get me them bills back?"

"It might," the doctor said. "It could put you into a recession and the bills will drop down and out. My advice is to make sure you wear panties for some extra security."

In the wee hours of the morning, a guard walked me to my car. A fellow Irishman, he kept the pleasantries going for the three blocks until we got to my dented Volkswagen bug. As I was about to get in the car, I could see by his serious expression that something was troubling him.

"Is anything wrong?" I asked.

He shuffled a bit. "Well, I was wondering if you might be coming back again tomorrow?"

"Sure. I'll be here for the rest of the week."

He gently took my hand. "You seem like a nice lass, so won't you please take my advice and run like hell? Find another job. This one will turn you sour as an old lemon."

I didn't take his advice until a few years later when I was beyond sour and getting into downright bitter. I transferred to a posh ER where none of the patients carried semi-automatic weapons or kept their money or food items hidden in unorthodox places.

Still and all, I wouldn't have missed those few years in the war zone for anything. I think you have to be an ER nurse to fully understand that.

NORMA

"I entered nursing in 1955, but really, I'd been a nurse since the age of four when I began looking at the pictures in my mother's nursing textbooks.

"When I turned thirteen, my grandfather told me that I had many career choices. I asked what they were, and he said, 'Why, you can be a wife and mother, a waitress, or a secretary!'

"The difference between nursing of the fifties and sixties and modern nursing is that nowadays we no longer practice nursing—we do tasks. We no longer nurse the patients—we just give the medicines and run the equipment.

"The attitudes of the physicians have historically been a problem and they remain a problem. For example, a physician who felt it necessary to have a physical division between nurses and doctors, designed our trauma center. The doctor's side is a large, fully equipped office with coffee machine, couches and tables, a TV, and huge windows overlooking a courtyard garden.

"On the other side of the wall is a small counter with three rolling chairs where the nurses are supposed to work—no windows, no couches, no coffee machine, and no TV. We do, however, have a set of lights over the counter. When the physicians need a nurse, they press a button and the lights blink on the nurse's side of the wall. The doctors chose to use red light bulbs to get the nurse's attention. I *believe there is some significance in that—press a button, flash the red lights, here comes the nurse/whore to tend to their whims.*

"The nurses have repeatedly asked that the dividing wall be taken down and the red lights be replaced. The physicians refuse, giving no explanation other than that's the way they like it.

"The hospital administration caters to them. If a doctor makes one complaint about a nurse, be it floor nurse or the director of nursing, that nurse is never to be seen again. It's like the Dark Ages."

1960 Arkansas

I was catching up on my charting when I heard a low whimpering behind me. I turned in the direction of the sound and sucked in my breath.

Standing alone in the hallway that went to the ambulance bay was a young child wearing nothing but what had once been a pair of bathing trunks. Burned from the top of his head to his toes, I focused on the long red and black flaps of skin and muscle hanging from each of his armpits.

It was probably less than one second that I sat there trying to make sense of what I was seeing, but it seemed like forever. I certainly don't remember jumping over the desk, although I was later told that's what I did.

I recall wondering how I was going to pick him up, but when I got behind him, I cried in relief to see that his backside wasn't burned. I managed to scoop him into my arms, touching only unburned skin. When I ran into the main room, the doc and the other nurse took one look at my armload, froze for a second and then went into action.

"Where are the parents?" the nurse asked, already checking his airway.

"He just appeared in the back hallway," I said. "There was no one with him."

She told me to find the parents, so I went back to the hallway, but it was empty. Out in the ambulance bay, I found an old station wagon with a man slumped over the wheel. I knocked on the window, but he didn't respond, so I opened the door. The man was mumbling, making no sense.

I'd seen various degrees of hysterical shock, but never anything like what I had before me. Appalling visions went through my mind of the child realizing his father was incapable of helping, then getting out of the car and walking the length of the hallway in order to help himself.

"Are you that boy's father?"

The man didn't answer so I pulled him from the car and more or less carried him into the hospital. As soon as he saw his son in the treatment room, his legs went out from under him.

I sedated him right there on the floor. When his breathing slowed and he could talk, he related what had happened in salvos of two or three words at a time.

It had been a day set aside for time with his only child. They'd gone fishing that morning then gone home to grill their catch on the backyard barbecue. He lit the coals and realized he'd poured in too much lighter fluid. Panicking, he kicked the barbecue into a bare section of the yard. At that moment, the child rounded the corner of the house and ran directly into the flames.

We admitted the boy with third degree burns over seventy percent of his body. His father was admitted for shock. For three days the staff worked under a blanket of depression while we listened to the child's screams every time they changed his dressings. The father heard them too, and as soon as the child began shrieking, his screams overtook his son's and drowned them out.

The fourth day brought an ominous silence. We prayed to hear those screams again, and grew depressed when we didn't. The boy died that night, and the father was released to attend to the details of his burial.

Two days later, I was sitting at the same desk by the door when the wail of the ambulance's sirens propelled me out of my chair. Call it premonition, but the second I opened the bay doors and saw the ambulance, I thought of the father and how he'd looked that day. That uncanny sixth sense which belongs to every nurse, told me exactly who was in the back of the rig DOA with a self-inflicted gunshot to the head.

1961 Arkansas

The B's were a prominent family in Arkansas. The family money and power had been handed down father-to-son for generations, until one of the sons failed to produce an heir. Rather than stop the greased chute of wealth, his wife secretly arranged to adopt an infant boy.

The go-between warned them that the baby's father was a convicted murderer and a drug addict, and the mother was in a mental institution for the criminally insane. The adoptive mother said it wouldn't matter because if the child were raised properly, his genetic make up would be of no consequence.

The boy—I'll call him Elvis, a popular name at the time—grew up handsome, intelligent, and, completely psychotic. Throughout his teens, we saw him in the ER at least once a week for either drug overdoses or injuries he'd sustained from some wild behavior or other.

When he was nineteen, he drove his motorcycle through the ER's doors to the trauma room where he crashed and broke his leg. At twenty, he ate a bicycle for the hell of it. It took him almost a year. Every six weeks, we posted the x-rays of his intestines on the light boxes then had contests to see who could identify the most bicycle parts.

On his twenty-first birthday, Elvis came in and sat quietly in the waiting room. Every time I went out to get a patient, he would smile and wave. At first I thought he'd come in because it was the one place he felt safe and calm, but the longer he sat there wearing that stupid grin, the more I got to thinking that he was there to do mischief.

According to the patient sitting next to Elvis, the birthday boy began whistling Happy Birthday as he calmly took out his hunting knife, unzipped his fly and cut off his own penis. As he went into shock, he put the appendage in a paper sack and told the clerk to bring it back to the nurses.

One year later, Elvis walked into an emergency room in Little Rock dressed in Japanese robes he'd found in some costume shop. In full view of the clerk, he unrolled a mat, opened a case holding a sword, and committed hara-kiri.

Needless to say, Elvis's adoptive mother changed her mind regarding the good upbringing vs. the bad gene theory.

1962 Arkansas

The rattletrap of a truck coasted into the ER parking lot and came to a stop twelve feet from the front door. I put away the remainder of my lunch and waited to see what would emerge. We'd been slow all morning, so I was hoping for a little excitement.

Dressed in a worn cotton dress, her lack of teeth and personal grooming told me the woman was from the back woods. She looked to be about fifty years old, though I would have bet money she wasn't a day over twenty-four.

She went around to the passenger side of the truck, hesitated for a moment, then opened the door and reached in to grab a squirming burlap sack. Hoisting it over her shoulder, she looked to me for direction. "Where to go? My boy got hisself a bad broke arm."

I led her to the treatment room where she threw the sack down on the floor and stood back cussing, holding onto her shoulder, which was bleeding profusely. I leaned forward to check the wound then pulled back, certain the teeth marks were human. Whoever was in the bag had taken a good chunk out of her. I offered a gauze pad soaked with liquid soap that she refused despite my warnings that human bites usually became infected.

Turning my attention to the bag, I saw that the end had been tied off tight with the type of rope used to tie hogs.

"Don't you be messin' with that business in there, ma'am," the woman warned. "Git the doctor-man. The boy's afeared of men folk."

Ignoring her warning, I untied the bag. The overpowering stench of urine and feces wafted over me, giving me pause. I covered my nose and mouth and yanked the bag off the boy.

Because inbreeding was common in the backwoods, I expected something half-human with maybe two heads. Instead, I saw a fairly normal looking eight-year-old caked with layers of filth, although his eyes held all the ferociousness of a wild animal.

I moved closer to get a better look at his fractured arm, all the while speaking in hushed tones. I was just a few inches from him when the boy reared back and growled like a mad dog that means business.

"Git back ma'am," the mother warned, pulling on my arm. "He gonna bite you bad."

I sent the mother to the waiting room with assurances that I would get the 'doctor-man' for her son. When I returned to the treatment room, I found the boy cowering under the gurney, the canvas bag pulled over his head.

Keeping a respectful distance, I asked if his arm hurt, and if he could tell me what happened. The boy began slapping the floor, and made a series of grunting noises. That was when I realized he was deaf.

When the doctor tried to pick him up, the child screeched and literally climbed up the walls. It took six people to subdue him. The amount of sedation we gave this ninety-pound child could have felled a two hundred pound man.

While they set the child's arm, I went out to the truck and found his mother asleep in the back. I gave her a cup of coffee and the sandwich from my lunch.

"How do you communicate with him at home?" I asked.

"We don't do nothin', 'cept to feed him."

"Have you ever tried teaching him basic hand signs or how to read and write?"

She shook her head. "I tried once, but my old man 'bout went crazy mad. He got a temper on him all right, like when he found out the boy were dumb, I thought he were gonna kill me. The old man took that boy and put him in a cage out in the shed. He still keep him out there, 'cept when he works him in the fields."

I was horrified, but bit my tongue reminding myself that she was from a culture and a way of life very different from my own. I doubted I'd ever be able to understand it.

Lots of child abuse and incest went on in those backwoods communities back then. It was never talked about, but many of the children, both male and female, were sexually abused by their fathers and brothers. Most folks turned a blind eye, and the mothers never did anything about it, more than likely because they themselves had been abused growing up. Child abuse of whatever nature was a normal rite of passage in those parts.

Still, I talked to the mother for an hour about how she couldn't allow the child to live in a cage like an animal. I told her he deserved to have a chance in life, and there were things that could be done to help him—that there were many deaf children who led normal lives.

She kept nodding and saying she'd tried to help her son, but the old man had beaten her every time. She'd begged him to let her bring the boy to her married sister in Nashville so that he could get some proper help, but he always refused, saying it weren't nobody's business but his own.

I asked if she'd be willing to drive the boy to her sister's if we gave her money for gas. It took her a long time to answer, but she finally said she would.

I called the police who were not at all interested in helping the woman out. Truth be told, I got the distinct impression most of them agreed with the way the father had handled the situation.

I marched back into the ER and got everybody to give me as much money as they could. I guess the cops got to feeling guilty, because they showed up with gas and oil for the truck. We gave the mother some pain pills and a sedative for the boy, and sent them on their way.

The hospital was on the interstate, so that when people went out the driveway, there were only two ways to go—right took you to Tennessee, left went to the backwoods.

As she drove away, we all went outside to see what she would do. At the top of the driveway, she turned off the motor and sat there staring at the interstate for close to thirty minutes. When she started the car, she inched to the stop sign, and turned left.

I was the only one who was surprised.

1962 Florida

I started out the shift feeling mean as an old mule. First of all, it was a holiday weekend *and* a full moon and there were only two of us assigned to work that night. Secondly, the other nurse on duty that night was a rookie, and dumb as dirt besides.

If those two reasons weren't enough to justify being cranky, I'd had almost no sleep the night before because I'd been tending to one of the local farmers. For whatever reason, a lot of the farmers suffered from urinary retention and word got around that I could painlessly catheterize a man faster than they could tie a hog. It got so that I had to keep a stock of sterilized catheters at home. It wasn't unusual to get at least one call a week, usually in the wee hours of the morning, from one of the farmer's wives begging me to come over and relieve her husband.

I never asked for payment, but within the week I'd find a few new chickens in the yard, or a new piglet in the pen. On the front porch would be a jar of preserves or maybe a pie.

So there I was in what we loosely termed an emergency room, trying to humor myself into a better frame of mind, when a cop car pulls up with the lights and sirens still going. Two cops jumped out and pulled a man in handcuffs from the back. His pants were torn up the middle to his knees, and there was blood caked on his legs. Judging from the rough way the cops were handling him, I knew he must have done something really bad.

They handcuffed him to a gurney in one of the back rooms and left him in the care of the rookie nurse. Out at the desk, the cops told me the patient was a two-bit crook who'd broken into a farmhouse and point-blank killed the whole family—two parents and their three kids. The neighbor heard the shots and called the police. During a foot chase, the murderer had been shot in both legs.

While the cops put a call into the dispatcher, I went back to check on the prisoner. Upon entering the room, the air was so thick with sexual tension, it could have been a strip joint. The nurse had unbuttoned the top of her uniform so that her cleavage almost obscured her stethoscope. I glared at her, but the dumb cluck didn't get the message. Instead, she and the thug started talking flirty-dirty.

The man was a sweet-talker, I'll give him that. In the time it took me to check his wounds and set up an instrument tray, he had extracted the nurse's name, address, marital status (single and living alone) and phone number.

When I looked up, the nurse was rubbing his arms and giggling.

"What the hell are you doing?" I snapped, jerking her away. I wanted to throttle her. "This creep has just murdered a whole family in cold blood."

"But his arms hurt," she pouted. "Those cuffs are on too tight. We've got to get the circulation moving to his hands."

I stared at her in disbelief. The idea that his being a murderer had no consequence in her mind, left me so disgusted I stormed out to the main desk—a stupid move on my part.

About five minutes later, a simple equation went through my mind that literally shot me out of my chair: Young, dumb nurse with raging hormones, add handsome, sweet-talking con-man/murderer. Add to that the fact that the cops routinely left the keys to the handcuffs with the attending nurse, and you come up with a major disaster.

I wasn't ten feet from the door when the snaky bastard slithered out of the room holding a small pistol that he'd hidden in his boot. I wondered if he'd killed the other nurse and if he had, how the hell was I going to handle the whole unit by myself for the rest of the night. Not entirely logical thinking, but then again I also thought I was in total control of the situation. Even when he grabbed me by the throat and dragged me into the main room, the gun pointed at my temple, I was irritated by the thought of the paperwork he was creating for me.

Now, it is a little known fact that ER nurses are proficient at cussing. If provoked, they are capable of uttering some of the vilest gutter language in existence. As for myself, I can swear harder and better than any sailor, whore, Hell's Angel or truck driver on earth.

The disruption of my day with this piece of no account shit pissed me off so bad that I blew my top. Knocking his arm away, I got up in his face and screamed a string of swear words I guarantee he'd never heard come out of a woman's mouth ever before. I know this for a fact, because that man literally stumbled backward, shock written all over his face.

And thank God for my dirty mouth, because it so distracted the jerk, the cops were able to grab him from behind without anybody getting killed.

1969 Florida

It was the second night of an August full moon and insane things were happening outside. Our youngest state trooper, a good man with only one year on the force, brought in a guy he'd spent two hours talking down from the ledge of a building. Most of the other troopers would probably have helped the man jump, but the rookie still had a few ounces of compassion left in him.

We held the jumper in the ER, but while we were waiting for the psychologist to come in and admit him to the psych unit, he escaped. Two hours later he came in DOA, the chain he'd used to hang himself still around his neck.

The rookie cop was so torn up over it that I sat with him trying to lighten him up. I plied him with coffee and pie, kidding him about the ten pounds he'd put on in the six months he'd been married.

That loosened him up enough to get him joking about how he'd grown too fat for his bulletproof vest, and the chief wasn't happy about having to order a new one.

An hour later, the radio dispatcher announced that a cop had been shot and was on his way to us. Of course it turned out to be the rookie, and of course, the shot had been through his chest where the vest should have been. We worked for an hour to save him, but the bullet had done too much damage.

You'd think that things couldn't get any worse, but they did. The trooper's new bride had been listening to the police scanner and came into the ER thinking that the dead trooper was somebody *else's* husband, and she was going to help the new widow. I was the one to tell her it was her own husband.

Two hours after the trooper died, a middle-aged couple came in with their unconscious eighteen-year-old son. They explained that over dinner, he and his nineteen-year-old brother had gotten into a violent argument and the younger son had retreated to his room. An hour later, his mother found him in bed, completely unresponsive.

We examined him six times over and found no signs of violence. The tests for common poisons and drugs all came back negative. With not much to go on, we did a series of skull x-rays.

When we put the films on the light boxes, what jumped out at us was a long, thin metal object that went from the front of his skull to the back. We looked from the x-rays to the boy lying on the gurney.

"Damn it," said the doctor, "What numbskull left their pen on the x-ray table?"

I went to the x-ray department and looked all over for the pen but found nothing. I was walking across the room, squinting at the x-rays on the light boxes, when I realized what we were looking at.

"Oh my God!" I said, "That isn't a pen, it's a nail file."

And that's exactly what it was. Apparently the younger boy had gone to his room and fallen asleep. The older brother snuck in, pulled down his brother's lower eyelid, and shoved a six-inch nail file through his brain without leaving a trace.

When questioned by the police, the brother said he'd read about someone using this method to murder someone in a dime store crime novel, and thought he'd give it a try.

1970 Florida

A drunk driver killed my only child when she was nineteen. It changed my life forever, but not in the way most people would think. To me death is okay for everybody no matter what age they are. I don't get overly emotional over SIDS babies or two-year-olds or teenagers dying. I never think, *Oh what a shame this baby died so young.*

I also don't believe in fate. When my daughter was killed, my mother-in-law said she'd died for a reason, and someday, if we were blessed, we would realize what the reason was. That turned me off more than anything, because I don't believe it for a second. I believe there are accidents and people die. There is disease and people die. We live and we die. The length of time between birth and death is insignificant.

Because of my daughter's death, I have always had an affinity with people who lose their children. Sometimes I get involved with these families on a very emotional level. Those are the cases that haunt me.

It was August in south central Florida and hotter than blazes. Most people in the area were poor farmers who could barely keep themselves and their families alive with what they produced, let alone having luxuries like telephones or air conditioning. Very few of them could even afford to own a car unless it was something they built themselves.

It was from one of these outlying farms that we got a three-year-old girl who had been bitten on the leg by a coral snake while playing in her yard. The mother had been inside feeding her six-month old when she looked out the window and saw her little girl reaching for the brightly colored snake. Her warning scream came too late.

In the hottest part of the day, she carried both children for the better part of a mile to the nearest neighbor's house. When she could go no farther, the injured girl had to walk. The mother knew it was the wrong thing to do but she couldn't carry both children and not pass out from the heat.

We worked like the dickens to save that child, but she died anyway. I recall sitting and talking to the mother, but no matter what I said, she was smothered under a huge pile of guilt.

Later, the other nurses offered to take the child to the morgue, but I couldn't allow anyone else to touch her. Instead of undressing her, putting on the toe tag and taping down her arms, I bundled her up in the nicest blanket I could find. When the orderly brought in the morgue cart, I tried, but I couldn't put her on it, so I carried her to the morgue.

The normal procedure was to place the body on one of the slabs, cover it with a sheet and make a notation on the sign-in board for the coroner, but when I set her down, I couldn't pull that sheet over her face. I left her wrapped up with her little face showing.

Then I had a problem with turning off the lights. I couldn't leave that baby alone in the dark. I kept thinking, *No, it's too dark for her in here.*

I backed out the door with that little china doll face in my mind, and to this day it has never left me.

1975 Southern California

The Civil Rights Movement came, planted a few soul food restaurants and was gone. However, I am here to let you know that racial discrimination was and is very much alive and thriving in this so-called land of the free.

In the sixties, I'd marched for civil rights and wore peace signs embroidered on my clothes right along with everyone else. I'd also worked in some of the most racially prejudiced places on earth with some of the worst dyed-in-the-wool bigots you'd ever want to meet.

So, when I took a temporary ER job in Southern California, the liberal peace and love civil rights capital of the world, I thought it was going to be a "groovy love all your brothers and sisters regardless of color and creed" sort of atmosphere.

That idea was blown all to hell the day the ambulance brought in a giant of a black man into our ever-so-groovy California ER.

The man was massive—six-feet-seven inches tall, and over three hundred fifty pounds of pure muscle. He was so big, that when the ambulance driver and cops pulled the stretcher off the rig, they couldn't lift it. It stayed about a foot off the ground.

The cops reported that the patient was "badly hurt," so I directed them to the trauma room, and called for the doctor. As we were rolling across the main section of the unit, the doctor walked into the room and held up a hand to stop us.

"Don't you dare mess up my trauma room with that nigger," he said in his most authoritative, nasty tone. "Put him over there in the corner where he belongs." He pointed to the gurney in the corner by the utility sinks.

I may not have believed what I'd heard come out of that doctor's mouth, but the man on the stretcher sure did, because he broke through his leather straps like they were made out of crepe paper. I'd never seen anyone do that before except in old horror movies.

That man got right up in the doctor's face and grabbed for his throat with a hand that was bigger than the doctor's whole head.

The doctor jumped on top of the counter screaming like a girl. "For God's sake, do something! He's going to kill me!"

The cops just stood there. I thought they didn't react because they wanted to teach the racist bastard a lesson, but that thought was dashed when one of them said, "What do you want me to do to him doc? I've already unloaded my gun into him twice."

We all focused back on the patient and realized he was bleeding profusely from what looked like a hundred bullet holes. At that moment, the man took another step toward the doc and fell through the glass cabinets where we kept the specialty instruments.

Two other nurses and I started to help him, but the doctor jumped down from the counter and shoved us away. "Just leave him alone," he shouted, "He'll bleed to death in a few minutes."

I desperately wanted to call the cops, but they were already there. Worse yet, they were in agreement with the doctor's method of treatment. I tried to do CPR and was immediately yanked to my feet by one of the cops. He shoved a finger in my face and warned me to back off.

Horrified, I watched the man bleed to death right there on the floor of the ER. They wouldn't even let me hold his hand. It was one cold way to die.

1977 Las Vegas

Ms. Sweet was a supervisor nurse. True to her name, she was one of those rare human beings who had a smile and a kind word for everyone. No matter how hot or messy it was in the ER, she always wore a proper starched white uniform with long sleeves and white stockings. More importantly, she was always there when you needed her.

It was a slow September night when one of our ambulances was dispatched to a downtown address. I recognized the address as belonging to a certain attorney's office and made what was probably one of the original lawyer jokes—something about how seeing as he was an attorney, maybe he'd choked on his own slime.

When the paramedics called in, they described an unconscious, unresponsive middle-aged woman who wasn't breathing very well. They were unable to pass an endotracheal tube because her airway was partially obstructed by swelling. She had a rhythm, but it was erratic.

When the stretcher came in, you could have knocked us over with a feather—the patient was none other than Ms. Sweet, and the attorney was her husband.

He told us that one-minute she was talking to him, and the next, she fell unconscious to the floor. The thing that struck everyone as odd was the fact that he showed no emotion whatsoever.

His insistence that he be present in the trauma room, we chalked up to his being an attorney, but the entire time we worked on Ms. Sweet, he stood over the doctor, methodically taking notes and asking detailed questions about everything we were doing. Never once did he ask if his wife was going to survive, and he never tried to talk to or touch her. All he wanted to know was the technical minutia, like what size tube we were using, and what IV solutions were hung.

Of course, the questions were meant to be threatening, and although he had an ominous presence, I allowed him to stay because, unlike most other ER personnel, I firmly believe the patient's family has a right to see what actually takes place behind the closed doors of an ER.

I used my famous crash sheers—the ones that had cut through hundreds of bootlaces and tight jeans—to rip through Ms. Sweet's blouse and slacks. The clothes fell away revealing multiple bruises, old and fresh. Around her neck were obvious bruises, synonymous with those we saw on certain murder victims.

"Oh my God, she's been strangled!" I said, stating the obvious.

Her husband instantly leapt at me, shaking his fist in my face. "People go to prison for making false statements like that! I'll make sure you come to regret that remark!"

He then tried psyching us out by writing down everyone's name in his little notebook. We all thought he was potentially physically dangerous, so nobody said another word until we got Ms. Sweet intubated and up to ICU.

It was touch and go for Ms. Sweet. I went to see her every day, and finally, when she was lucid and could talk, we discussed what had happened. I told her she couldn't allow her husband to beat her again, and that she should get a restraining order and divorce him.

My advice had little effect, because Ms. Sweet resigned before she was even discharged from the hospital. Within the month, she'd moved to Arizona with her husband, and we never heard another word from her. A couple of us wrote letters, but they were always returned, unopened.

About two years later, on one of those rare slow nights in ER when the nurses sit around swapping ER horror stories, a recently hired nurse described a woman who'd arrived at her former ER one night, dead on arrival.

In the ensuing brouhaha, it was brought to light that her husband had beaten her to death. Because he was an attorney, he'd managed to arrange things with the DA's office so that he was never indicted.

"The real bummer part of the story," the nurse said, "Is that this woman was an ER nurse."

We all froze and went silent, because we knew. I asked if she remembered the dead nurse's last name.

"Sure," she said, "Sweet—it's a hard name to forget."

1981 Florida

The ER nightmares were wearing me down, so I was glad to be working ICU for a change. Besides, there was a certain comfort in having the elements of violence and surprise removed from my patient population.

My assignment was good old boring fare of end stage renal failure, and standard issue cerebral vascular accidents. The ICU patients were predictable—they either got better or died. They were clean. They were quiet. Here there were no drunks smelling of sewage and pissing on my shoes. ICU was where things were nice and slow. Everything was planned out for twelve hours in advance; no one's life was depending on my split-second actions and decisions.

I was so laid back, that even when the charge nurse dumped a fifth patient on me at mid-shift, I didn't complain. Used to having twenty-five or more very angry patients in an ER waiting room, five patients in ICU was nothing.

I took report from the ER nurse, trying hard to keep the smug attitude out of my voice, although I did make some snotty comment about having only four sweet-smelling, clean and manageable patients who were actually pleasant human beings.

The ER nurse sniffed defensively and kept right on with report. "Ever hear of X food company?"

Who hadn't heard of them? X food products were as well known around the world as Coca-Cola.

"Well, this is Mrs. X," she continued, "wife of the original X foods mogul. She's had a massive stroke and isn't expected to live more than a few days, but we have to make it look like we struggled valiantly to bring her back from the dead, which is why she's coming to ICU instead of going to the general medical floor."

She gave report then added as an afterthought, "And by the way, the family is a bit eccentric. The old lady's doctor says to let them have whatever they want."

"Eccentric like how?"

"You know, eccentric like rich people."

I sighed. I did know. After all my years in the ER, dealing with the wealthy, arrogant, entitled population was more trying and exhausting than handling the vilest of street bums.

There was only one private room available in the ICU, and Mrs. X's name was on it. Before I could even push the ventilator into the room, the lesser ranks of the X family servants were replacing the hospital bedding with down mattress pads and Egyptian cotton sheets. Every available space was filled with sprays of designer flowers, and works of original art were hung on the walls.

Finally, Mrs. X arrived on a gurney with all the pomp and circumstance of Cleopatra sailing down the Cydnus River on her barge—albeit a Cleopatra with respirator, three IVs, cardiac monitor, urinary catheter, nasogastric tube, suction canisters, arterial and pulmonary lines.

In procession were the heirs—two ungracefully aging daughters, one balding, paunchy son, and a gaggle of grandkids in sporty designer wear. Bringing up the rear was the faithful family retainer who had orders to stay close to the patient at all times.

The whole scene grated on my nerves, but crowd control proved easy: I sent the grandchildren away at once, much to their relief. At the first sight of blood and mucous, the retainer turned green and had to be wheeled away. This left the three direct descendents to the task of deathwatch.

With critical care equipment in place and calibrated, I was about to begin my physical and neurological assessments, when there was a soft knock at the door. With a command from the elder daughter the door flew open and several racks, heavily laden with all manner of clothing, were wheeled in.

The gowns and dresses were divided into groups: Armani to the right of the rack, Dior to the left, and Chanel hung sleeve-to-sleeve with the furs and cashmere capes. The bottoms and tops of the racks were covered with expensive shoes, purses, and hats.

Next to invade the room were three women carrying professional cases. At once they attended to my patient's hair, nails and make-up.

I pulled back to take in the scene. A comatose old woman lying in a critical care bed, intubated and hooked to a ventilator, plastic tubes coming from every orifice, most of them draining odious fluids of brown, yellow, red or green. Surrounding her were all the accoutrements of a beauty queen about to enter her last contest.

"I'll want to dress my mother for the dinner hour," her daughter said, waving an imperial hand. "I'll need help removing some of these tubes."

"The dinner hour?" I repeated.

"Yes," she said, eyeing me up and down. "Civilized people dress for dinner, you know."

"I'm sure they do, but not in ICU. First of all, your mother won't be eating, and there's no way you can dress your mother in one of those gowns while she has all that equipment in and on her. Not only would the gown be ruined with blood or some other body fluid, but removing any of those tubes could very well cause your mother to die."

Unruffled, the daughters conferred for a few minutes then asked if I would please remove their mother's patient gown.

Because I'd been told to give them what they wanted, I did so, curious as to how they were going to deal with the matter of the tubes. The younger daughter chose a gown with beads woven into the bodice, and held the material up to the blue respirator tubing to see if it clashed.

It clashed.

The elder daughter chose the ecru Chanel with gold braid and laid it carefully on top of her mother's body, tucking it under her here and there. The son then rolled a pair of silk stockings over his mother's edematous legs and managed to fit her swollen feet into a pair of matching evening pumps.

By the time they'd finished, the old lady looked like the Queen Mother going to a coronation.

For the three days she lived, the old dame had her frocks changed twice a day for the luncheon and dinner hour. The ritual was a pain in the ass to deal with, moving the tubes around and making sure nothing dribbled or spilled, but I have to admit that it was a rather refreshing break from the ER.

KATHLEEN HOLLOWED
Washington Hospital, Burn Center

"I have been a nurse for twenty years, nineteen of them spent working in burn units. When I graduated from nursing school, I didn't have a car. My parents told me I had to get a job and I had to figure out how to get there. So, I picked the hospital job that was on my bus line—the adult and pediatric burn unit.

"Burn nursing is probably one of the most difficult jobs you can do. The nurse has to have an enormous knowledge base since burns affect all systems of the body. Plus, the patients are as down as they could possibly be, and the nurse has to help them become a functioning part of the world again.

"After six years of watching six and seven-year-old kids die, I kind of lost it. I took time off, and then went to the OR. It took about a year of doing mindless work for me to realize that I wanted more of a challenge—I needed to get my hands dirty. That was when I took a job in the Washington, D.C. burn center."

September 11, 2001
Washington, D.C.
In the middle of running around doing errands, an announcement came over the car radio that one of the

World Trade towers was on fire. The announcer stopped in the middle of his statement and said, "Oh my God, a plane just flew into the second tower!"

As I pulled into the hospital parking lot, I overheard someone say that the Pentagon was on fire. I remember thinking, *Okay, so we'll probably get a couple of patients.*

I was walking to my office when Dr. Jordan, the Burn Center Director, told me to get into my scrubs immediately and meet him in MedStar, which is our trauma unit.

When I got to MedStar, it was Dr. Jordan, Dr. Jeng, the nurse practitioner, and me. The nurse practitioner left me to handle the situation while she went upstairs and got things ready in the acute burn area. At this point all I was thinking was, *They're going to come in and we're going to intubate them, get lines into them and throw them into secondary triage.*

As soon as a patient came off the MedStar helicopter, I was to mark off exactly where the burns were on a diagram of the human body. Then I'd figure out what percentage of the body was burned, using the Rule of Nines—this is a mathematical formula that helps calculate the total body surface area involved in burns. It tells us exactly how much fluid we need to give the patient for the fluid resuscitation.

At 10 a.m. we got our first patient in Bay 1. Interestingly enough, he didn't have to be intubated, and his burns were only about twenty-four percent—arms, hands and face. He kept repeating, "Call my wife, call my wife," so I took the wife's number and asked Decedent Affairs to contact her. I wanted to calm him down, but we all had visions of hundreds of patients coming to us, so I couldn't really talk to him for very long, since the whole idea was to get them in, do our thing, and get them upstairs.

I moved to Bay 2 and saw something I'd never seen in all my twenty years of burn nursing. The patient's face was so severely burned, that his eyes had been burned open. He was already being intubated, so I did his burn diagram, completed the formula, secured it to his blanket and moved to Bay 3.

Mrs. H was a local civilian woman who had at least fifty-five percent burns plus a large gaping wound in her abdomen. That snapped everybody into instant trauma awareness. In other words, we suddenly realized these people might have more injuries than just burns. I quickly figured out the formula for her and went back to Bay 1 where Mrs. K had already replaced the man who'd been asking for his wife. Mrs. K was one of the worst bad luck cases I've ever heard of—9/11 was her second day on the job. When we walked into the room, Drs. Jordan and Jeng and I took one look at her and then at each other, and gave a collective sigh. She had full-thickness burns to both hands, which meant her fingers would not be salvageable.

In Bay 2 the man without eyelids had been replaced by a young black woman with sixty-five percent burns and major inhalation injuries. She had inhaled an enormous amount of jet fuel, so I wasn't surprised when she died a week later of pulmonary complications.

The burn patients were all conscious when they came in, and that's because the body doesn't realize right away that it has been burned. It takes about forty-five minutes to an hour before there's a fluid shift that causes swelling, which can compromise the patient's airway. It's very rare that a burn patient goes into burn shock in that first hour. If the burn is third degree, the nerve endings have all been destroyed, so there is no pain. Most of the Pentagon victims were third degree.

People always ask how I can stand the smell of burned flesh, and I can honestly say that I don't notice that smell. Maybe I'm immune to it, but the smell I *did* notice that day was jet fuel. Every patient who came in had inhaled and swallowed jet fuel after the tanks exploded and deluged everyone.

With burns, you have to think in terms of the exact moment the injuries occurred. For example, what was the positioning of the body? How close or far from the fire or blast was the person? With the Pentagon patients, we figured that at the moment of impact, their mouths had probably been open in a gasp of surprise or a scream, and they got a blast of fuel in both airway and stomach.

All the patients except two had significant pulmonary injury. The other two had been positioned within the structure of the Pentagon in such a way that they did not take on that direct hit of fuel. What was really strange was that all of the survivors suffered back burns, but few injuries to the chest area, although their faces, arms and hands were burned.

When we finally sat down to study the diagrams the Pentagon gave us, we tried to figure out where the plane hit. Dr. Jordan spoke with each patient and asked questions about where they were and what position they'd been in at the moment of impact.

One of the patients was in the bathroom, although we told the press he was in the corridor because, well, we really didn't want to say he'd been taking his morning ritual in the men's room.

One of the men was in the Naval Command Center. What was interesting with him was that he was in an office cubicle with three other men when the plane hit. They were all close in proximity, with the one differing detail that our patient was the only one standing. The other three men, who were sitting only inches away, all died.

Some of the Pentagon survivors do talk about it, but I personally don't press the issue. I've done burns long enough to know burn patients don't like reliving the experience. Even though they were conscious when they came in, most of them didn't know what had happened. It wasn't until a few weeks later that they all remembered the initial impact of the jet. We had only one patient who wouldn't talk about anything that happened that day. He was total Army—wouldn't say a word until he personally got the okay from President Bush.

When these people were moved into secondary triage, it got very weird because we had no more patients coming in. Every time we'd hear sirens, we'd think they were bringing us patients, but they didn't. It was like, *Wait a minute, you mean this is it?* That made me sick to my stomach because I soon realized that probably hundreds of people were dead and we weren't going to get any more of them out.

In secondary triage, I made sure each patient was weighed and the dressings were all changed before Drs. Jordan and Jeng told us to start bringing them into surgery.

Normally we wouldn't perform surgery that quickly; we'd do the fluid resuscitation first and then wait forty-eight hours for the burn to declare itself. But being that we still weren't sure how many patients we were going to get, Drs. Jeng and Jordan opted to start excising the wounds immediately so as to get ahead of the game and cut away the burned tissues in hopes the body wouldn't notice yet that it had been burned. That way we might be able to avoid a lot of the shock issues. The patients went to the operating room two at a time, and for the rest of the day I floated between the operating room and the receiving units.

Normally, the military would transfer all their active duty burn patients to their burn facility in Texas, but nobody was allowed to fly, not even the military. When President Bush came in on Thursday morning, he made the statement to the families and patients that they were in the best possible burn center in the United States. So, of course, when the families were faced with the prospect of having their loved ones transferred to Texas, they balked.

They were like, "No way! You aren't sending my loved one to Texas. President Bush said this is the best place, so we're staying!"

I didn't watch TV or read a paper for a week. I went home at midnight, fell asleep, got up early and worked fifteen to sixteen hours, then went home and slept some more. The rest of the time I was doing hands-on care, taking care of the public relations, and worrying about Drs. Jordan and Jeng.

Lack of sleep became an issue for Drs. Jordan and Jeng to the point where the staff was extremely worried about them. I tried to guide them, acting more or less like their mom. I kept saying, "Look, you need to go to your room and sleep for a little bit." but they wouldn't listen. They operated until four or five every morning from September 11, through the weekend.

Dr. Jeng finally went home late Friday night. He had four young children so we had to press upon him that his kids would be anxious and upset about not seeing him.

Saturday morning he came back in to relieve Dr. Jordan who hadn't left at all.

On Monday, September 17, I went home at a decent hour and actually turned on the TV. I remember watching the whole thing for the first time. I've never been to one of the debriefings, although I think I did my own debriefing when I went to Florida at the end of October to speak about what happened that day. That was the first time I fully felt the tragedy of what had happened and cried.

Our last patient was discharged on December 17, 2001. I still see some of them when they come back for treatments. The Pentagon burn survivors are just that— survivors. They suffered horrific injuries and survived physically, but emotionally, I think they have a little more baggage to deal with than most.

For most of us it was a good experience. What I mean by that is we were the lucky ones because we got to help and do what we are good at.

Still, I don't feel like a hero. I did my job. Period. I think of it this way: this is what nurses do. Burn nurses do what they do for the love of the patients and because we know what the outcome would be without us.

JILL

"Sick and irreverent humor is my approach to nursing. Regardless of the situation, I'll be the one cracking jokes. When I started out, I was constantly reprimanded with the statement that humor doesn't belong in nursing. Personally, I believe the more humor in nursing the better.

"The black humor that comes out of ER is, by most normal standards, sick. I refer to these stories as 'location situations' because you have to know what it's like to work in an ER to fully understand what's so funny. I find it amusing that when I tell a funny ER story to a non-medical person without a sense of humor, they'll get this disgusted expression that says, 'You need professional help.'

"When I was younger, I thought I wanted to be a flight attendant. Then I got on my first airplane and hated it. So I figured if I flew, I'd have to take drugs, and that would have made it difficult to tend to the passengers without slurring. That was when I decided to be a nurse with a sense of humor.

"ER nurses aren't good at just one thing—we have to be good at everything. Because of that, you sometimes get warped by your own power. Then you either turn into one of those humorless nurses, or, you get to be twisted like me.

"The straight dope is that ER nurses have such a distorted view of people that if we didn't have the black humor button, we'd all commit suicide."

My shift is twelve minutes old when we get our first wonky code of the night. Lately, most of the codes have been strange, so I know we're two or three days away from a full moon. Tonight the great unwashed masses are gearing up, getting ready for the onslaught.

I study the road map of varicose veins on the eighty-nine-year-old object of our efforts and listen to the paramedic's report of how she had the misfortune of ending up in our ER as a full code. Despondent over the mashed turnips her nursing home serves daily for lunch, she decided to take matters in her own hands and throw herself off the second story balcony.

As if this weren't enough, the paramedics have opted to use the automatic chest compressor, affectionately known as 'Thumper.' Thumper is thumping away like mad, further crushing the old lady's already crushed ribs. All these factors tell me that her chances of surviving are zero, but because she is a friend of a friend of the administrator's second cousin's wife, we are obliged to put on a good show even though we all know perfectly well nothing we do to this elderly woman has a snowball's chance in hell of bringing her back to life. Or, as I like to tell people when they come in expecting miracles, "Dr. Frankenstein *used* to work here, but he quit a few months ago."

The code we run is all done by rote. Push in this drug, defibrillate, push in that drug, defibrillate, check the pupils, then the monitor. My mind wanders and finally focuses on Thumper's rhythm. Each compression makes a click, then a short psssht, and then there is a long, swooshy whissshhht with each forced breath from the ventilator.

For a few minutes we continue pouring in the drugs until Dr. D stops what he's doing and says, "Okay, can anybody think of what else we could possibly try here?"

Thoughtfully, I look at him and say, "Did you ever notice the beat on that thumper, Dr. D? It's the perfect rhythm for *Tea for Two*."

The respiratory therapist, the clerk, the doc and the other two nurses stop and listen. As if on cue, we all softly hum the refrain of *Tea for Two* with Thumper as the accompaniment.

There is no disrespect in this. We know we can't bring the old woman back so we might as well offer her a cheery send off. By the second chorus, we're all softly singing, and most of us are doing a little Fred Astaire soft shoe around the gurney as we work

A few minutes later, I'm tying a tag to the woman's toe when I catch the sounds of another stretcher rolling down the ambulance ramp. I peer out the round porthole window of the trauma room and see a large group of uniformed, gun-toting men surrounding a gurney that is headed for one of the other trauma rooms.

Ramon, our sarcastic department clerk, hands me the patient's chart. "A mummy's boy," he says and returns to his desk.

Discourteous as Ramon's one-line judgments may seem, I have learned to pay attention to them. His skills at profiling at a glance are astoundingly accurate.

Clyde is a prisoner from the maximum-security prison down the road. As the paramedic tells the story, Clyde and his archrival, Abdul, had been trying to kill each other with crude shivs fashioned out of toothbrushes. In the scuffle Clyde got shredded pretty good. According to the prison doctor's notes, he has lacerations to his face, chin, back, chest and buttocks. He is also missing an ear and two fingers.

Inside the trauma room, I can't see the patient through the six guards who surround him, so I know Clyde has to be a very bad dude. Clearing a path through the uniforms, I see that the prisoner's legs and arms are shackled to the steel frame of the gurney. When I get the full view of the patient, I am taken aback.

God bless those prison doctors. Most of them, I'm sure, are actually prisoners parading in lab coats. In all their misguided medicine, they have wrapped Clyde like a mummy, head to chained foot. They've used sixteen jumbo rolls of gauze if they've used one. The only things showing on the prisoner are his lips and one eye. Random spots of blood have managed to soak through the white gauze.

I cut a window through the gauze over the inner crook of his arm, find a nice vein and start a second intravenous line. I'm cleaning up when I notice the six by six square of white cardboard around which the IV tubing was wrapped.

Being who I am, my mind rushes toward the corner of Twisted Street and Peculiar Avenue. I take the permanent marker from my pocket and write in that famous and easily recognizable print:

got milk?

I then stick the sign to the end of Clyde's gurney.

Three of the guards start laughing and quickly leave the room. The other two guffaw as only big men can.

Clyde's eye wildly begins searching for the source of amusement. The mummy head lifts off the pillow. "What the fuck's so fucking funny?" the lips ask. His voice is low and gruff which somehow makes the innocent sign all the more perverse.

Unable to maintain any sort of serious guard-like demeanor, the two guffawing guards join their co-workers in the hallway.

"You assholes think a cut up dying man is funny?" The mummy's eye is going wild. "You gonna find out just how funny this is when we get back to the joint. Then we gonna see how hard you all laugh through slit throats."

The remaining guard takes out his handkerchief and wipes his eyes. "Take it away," he says, waving at the sign. He takes in the whole scene again and lets loose with outright laughter.

I remove the sign and go out to Ramon's desk only to find that the stack of incoming charts is close to twelve inches high. I look at my Timex and sigh.

It's after 9 p.m. The afternoon alcohol levels have dropped and those future patients are just now realizing that they've broken their leg in five places, or that the third degree burn they received when the barbecue blew up earlier is beginning to hurt.

I always think, *It took you four hours to realize this?* But, the blame has to be spread out equally because the sober straight arrows do it too. They'll go into congestive heart failure or have a heart attack about four in the afternoon, and I won't see them until six or more hours have passed. This is called denial.

A gurney rolls past me holding a man who looks pretty sober. Too sober. If I saw him at a party, I'd offer him a stiff drink. Ramon pushes a chart into my hand and nods once at the man with the empty eyes.

"I don't mean to be catty," Ramon whispers, "But this dude needs a helping hand."

The paramedics push the man toward the trauma room and I trail behind reading the EMS report. Mr. B, 57, has been deeply distressed for two months over the loss of his cat and alter ego, Mr. B Jr., 18.

Entering the room, one of the paramedics hands me a Playmate cooler. I don't need to open it to know that inside will be some body part that was recently attached to Mr. B Sr.

I turn up Mr. B's oxygen and take a blood pressure then gently roll down the head of the gurney so that he is laying flat. He struggles to sit up again, but I explain his blood pressure is low and I don't want him going into shock.

"Let me die!" Mr. B sobs. "I don't want to live without him."

"Mr. B," I say, getting serious, "you're talking about a cat, not your father or your son or even a spouse."

"He was all those things to me," he says, and I know that nothing I say is going to get through to him in his present state.

I turn up the IV drip rate and finish reading the report about how Mr. B took a butcher knife and chopped off his left hand, then clasped the same knife between his knees and attempted to saw off his right one. He'd just made a superficial cut when the UPS man showed up and called 911.

We don't call in Psych Services because Mr. B is going to be transferred to the microsurgery center in the city as soon as we get him stabilized. Their reattachment success rate is pretty good, although I'm not so sure how they do with hands.

I'm filling out the intra-facility transfer forms when a pale young man in a UPS uniform approaches, biting a fingernail.

"You're the one who called for assistance for Mr. B," I ask.

He nods. "How is he?"

"In need of massive amounts of microsurgery and psychotherapy, but otherwise he's okay."

The UPS man looks relieved and smiles as if this somehow lets him off the hook. He thanks me, starts to leave then turns back.

"I'm really happy he did it before he got the package. It would have bummed me out if he'd opened the package and then did this."

I appear sufficiently puzzled.

"The package I delivered was from the pet mortuary. It was his cat's ashes."

Because I need more information in order to complete the liability and insurance forms I return to Mr. B's bedside. Right after the question about what limb or body part was affected, I am required to ask how the loss of his hand will affect his life.

Mr. B bursts into tears anew and answers, "I liked petting my cat."

I finish up on Mr. B and hurry next door to the suture room. The chart is already in the door slot, signaling that Ramon is desperate to keep the pile at less than fourteen inches.

Before I go in, Ramon whispers, "Beauty queen on the scene."

Mr. O is twenty-four years old, drop-dead gorgeous, and very drunk. He is lying on a gurney cussing up a storm, flinging threats and insults at the nurses and doctors. When I approach, he immediately raises his annoying nasal voice and begins gesticulating. "You must save my face!" he hollers at the top of his lungs. "I'm a top model and I've got a *GQ* photo shoot first thing in the morning."

For being drunk he's pretty fast, because he has grabbed me by the front of my scrub top and is in my face before I can get out of range. I'm pretty sure you could get a good flame off the alcohol fumes on his breath were you to put a match to it.

"You have to fix it right!" Mr. O continues. "If you mess up my face, I'll sue you so hard you won't have shoes left to walk in! You better give me the best you've got."

I unhook his hands from my uniform, introduce myself and examine the one-inch laceration at his hairline. It's worthy of little more than two or three sutures, but it's clear his ego is calling for something more.

I decide to do what he's asked and give him the best that I've got. I summon Lily, one of the more overenthusiastic student nurses and ask her to prep the laceration for suturing.

Lily happily slaps on the Betadine, covering his hair, face, neck, and both ears with the sticky bright orange anti-bacterial solution. The solution easily washes off in the shower, but it is nonetheless shocking when a patient first sees himself with bright orange skin.

Next, Lily unwraps a hospital razor. Hospital razors look innocuous enough, but they are so sharp you could probably use one to castrate a rhino. Lily rests it on the GQ model's hairline.

Despite his mojito overdose, Mr. O feels the razor and starts to squirm. "Hey! What the hell are you going to do to my beautiful hair? You're gonna ruin me!"

I hold up the hand of medical authority and say in a bossy teacher sort of voice, "I'm sorry, but we need to shave around the area of the laceration. We don't want to risk infection."

GQ starts to protest, but I say, "Do you have any idea how much bacteria collects in the hair? The hair is a virtual Venus flytrap for bacteria. Have you ever seen a person whose face has been attacked by flesh-eating bacteria?"

I hold Mr. O's head still while Lily shaves the tiniest bit of hair away from the edges of the wound, as is our standard ER policy when managing scalp lacerations.

Lily spends a few minutes cleaning the wound again, making sure there are no stray hairs or dirt in the wound, when Mr. O slaps her hand away and pushes her hard enough to knock her down. Immediately, he begins exploring the wound with his dirty fingers.

I pull his hand away and tell him he is not to hit the nurses nor touch his wound. Undaunted, Lily springs to her feet and cleans his wound again.

We set up the suture tray and are trying to put a sterile paper drape over the laceration, when Mr. O turns mean and begins hurling insults at us and all those of our gender. When we don't react, he starts slapping at us. That doesn't get a reaction either.

However, it is when he begins to badmouth our profession that we decide we need to slather on another, thicker coat of Betadine—just to make sure we've got the bacteria covered.

By the time we are finished, Mr. O resembles a large naval orange with blue eyes and gleaming white teeth.

"Now," I announce, smiling, "we're ready for the doctor."

Dr. D enters the room. Startled, he takes a step back and stands speechless, staring at Mr. O's bright orange head. "Oh dear god," he sighs, then looks at us in the same way one might look at mischievous children who'd just put a toad in the sugar bowl. "What have you been doing to the nice patient?"

Lily and I smile innocently. "Why, we've adequately prepared the patient for you, doctor," Lily says.

Dr. D commences suturing the wound and tells Mr. O, "I'm doing my best work, so the scar will be invisible. Your hair is thick, so no one will notice the sutures. You'll be okay to do your photo shoot tomorrow.

"However—" Dr. D pauses to take a deep breath. "However, I, um, strongly suggest that as soon as you get home, you should just hop into the shower before looking in the mirror."

At this, Mr. O realizes something is amiss. Apprehensive, he asks, "Is there a mirror in here?"

"Nope, no mirrors," I say. "Sorry."

"How about a bathroom?"

Lily shakes her head. "I'm not sure."

Now Mr. O *knows* something is up. As soon as Dr. D gives him his follow-up instructions, he finds the bathroom. Lily and I count to two when we hear his long, high-pitched scream.

Mr. O's scream blends in with another coming from the trauma room. Through the door's porthole window I see a man in four point leather restraints. He is completely out of control.

Ramon steps in long enough to hand me a chart. "You should make sure he's been vaccinated for rabies," he says and disappears. The paramedic report states that after biting two of Macy's security guards, the patient was captured by police in the ladies sleepwear department. He has been brought to us for medical and psychiatric evaluation. Street drugs are definitely at work here.

As soon as I enter the trauma room, the first thought that comes to mind is of Dr. Hannibal Lecter in *Silence of the Lambs*. If we had one of those muzzle thingies that Hannibal wore over his mouth, we would use it now.

Our ersatz Hannibal is foaming at the mouth, taking huge bites out of the air. For as much as his restraints will let him, he is writhing around like a poisonous snake striking at anything that moves.

I stop three feet away from the gurney. He whips his head around, strains at his restraints, and chomps in my direction. I am not shocked to see that his teeth are filed to points, and his face is tattooed to resemble the head of a cobra.

"So, Dr. Lecter," I begin, "How's your day going?"

Hannibal curls his upper lip, to give the full view of his pointy fangs. His eyes roll all the way back and he is making strange animal noises. He spends a minute or two trying to get his head to swivel three hundred and sixty degrees, but soon tires of that and reverts to baring his teeth.

I see that someone living in a dream world has set up an IV tray. It strikes me that before anyone can get close enough to put an intravenous line into this guy, they will need a tranquilizer dart gun.

I am about to leave when it dawns on me that I would be remiss if I don't post a warning for the lab and x-ray techs who might try to undo his restraints. I am just about to tape the warning card to the end of his gurney when Dr. D comes in, takes the card out of my hand and reads aloud, "Do not release the Kraken."

He rips up the sign shaking his head, looks at me and sighs. "Honestly, Jill, what's wrong with you?"

"I can't help it," I say. "It's in my blood."

It's true. I'm constantly being called into the head nurse's office. I've been in there so many times, I've recently started giving her tips on how to redecorate.

It's getting late, and things have slowed down to the point where Dr. D is working on his taxes, Ramon is talking to his girlfriend who works at an all night doughnut shop, and I have time to restock the treatment rooms.

Walking right past the triage intake desk, a cute girl minces into our midst, wearing four-inch stiletto heels with the sexy straps, and a mini skirt cut up to her crotch. She's cradling her left hand as if it were a loved pet.

Despite the fake nails, breast implants, hair extensions, cheek implants, chin implant, chemical peel, nose job, colored contact lenses and the outfit, I have to admit, she is very cute. She is a walking damsel in distress, just ripe for rescuing.

"I need help," she says in a cute, helpless voice while shedding cute, fake tears.

Dr. D, who is young, virile, single and damned cute himself, is out of his chair like a shot, murmuring tender apologies for her pain.

Having secured male attention, she breaks into sobs that end in blubbering. "I was at this party?" She sniffles, flipping the made in China extensions over her shoulder. "And this stupid bozo opened the door just as I was reaching for the handle?"

Dr. D nods in complete understanding of the huge possibilities just under the front of her sweater.

"And . . . and he broke my nail and maybe the tip of my finger too!" She extends her hand carefully toward Dr. D as if it is going to fall off.

Dr. D touches her wrist, and she moans in a way that sounds more like she's having an orgasm than pain. This is more than I can bear, so I push Dr. D aside. "Let me get this straight. You broke your fake fingernail and you came to the ER?"

She nods. "There aren't any salons open at this time of night, so I figured since you guys can reattach people's legs and arms, you might have something that would work for a fingernail. Do you think you can help me?"

Dr. D, terrified of what I am going to say to this wonderful straight line opportunity, pushes me out of the way and cradles her arm. She leans against him, holding onto the lapel of his lab coat for support, and looks into his eyes.

When they turn to look at me, I see they have formed a bond and I am an intruder. Together, they bad vibe me right out of the room.

Dr. D medicates her with Tylenol for any possible physical or emotional pain, then, while Ramon and I watch, he sets her fake nail with Super Glue.

When the second coat of Luscious Licorice polish has dried over her medically reattached nail, I hand her the discharge instructions, which include Dr. D's home number at the bottom.

There must be some kind of major sports event on television, because we haven't had a patient come in for over an hour. Dr. T, who is presently paring his nails with suturing scissors, has replaced Dr. D. The other two nurses are asleep in treatment rooms eight and ten, Ramon is still talking to his girlfriend, and I'm plucking my eyebrows with surgical tweezers at the charting desk.

Esteban, one of our more fun orderlies, comes in with his boom box and plugs it in. As the first few beats rattle the x-ray boxes, Dr. T, who moonlights as a professional dancer, asks if I like to dance.

Unfortunately, I really do.

Gurneys are moved out into the hall, and the music is turned up louder. Thirty minutes later we've worked out a routine worthy of Michael Jackson before he turned white.

We are right at the point where Dr. T is supposed to lift me over his head, swing me around once and let me down into a backdrop. In a move so graceful I can barely believe it's me, I feel myself glide up and over his head.

It is here that I make the mistake of looking down. I freeze and lose my balance. To keep us from becoming our own next patients, I wrap my thighs round Dr. T's neck and hold on for dear life.

It is at this very moment that the head nurse enters the unit on her monthly Surprise Check-Up On The Nightshift rounds.

Dr. T staggers backward, toward her. I am above, facing her. Really, there is nothing I can do except smile and throw my arms over my head as though it is all part of ER's nightshift routine and this is a normal thing we do, like checking the crash cart.

Mouth set in a perfect 'O', she says nothing, backs up and closes the door behind her.

I know this means another trip to the principal's office, but that's okay—I've got an excuse ready—it's in my blood.

GLORIA

"I am a black woman, and I have seen it all in my seventeen years as a level one trauma center ER nurse on Chicago's Southside. Sometimes, the older white patients say they don't want a black nurse taking care of them. This area has a lot of old folks whose minds are still stuck on that nonsense. Can you believe they're still doing that shit? I always say, "Fine with me. I'll use my skills and knowledge somewhere else."

"If someone is calling me a nigger—and believe me, they do quite often—I won't take care of them at all. Lots of the patients here call the nurses bitches most of the time. It's so common that when they call me bitch, I respond, "Yes, may I help you?" Sometimes I think Bitch is my actual name.

My mother was an RN who used to let homeless people eat at our dinner table. The neighborhood kids teased us so bad, that to this day I can still hear them saying, "Your mama let them dirty old men eat at your table?"

But now I see myself doing the same thing. I see those people on the streets and I always give them money or food. My boyfriend says, "Gloria, why you give that man money? He could be on drugs."

And I say, "So what? He needs help. Our bellies are full, and here we are going home in a nice car to a warm house—these people got nothing."

That's what nurses are like. Nursing is a calling because not a lot of people can do the things we do. To see that trauma every day? It can really tear you up inside. People ask me all the time, "Gloria, how can you do them things you do?" I always say right back, "Somebody has to do it, and I'm the chosen one."

I was always afraid of the ER. I used to work on the regular medical floor, until the day I went down to see what the ER was like. There was so much blood everywhere, I thought, 'Oh my God, I'd probably faint if I worked here.'

But my girlfriend kept telling me to try it for a few days to see if I liked it. I did, and from the first day I worked there, I was in love and I have loved it ever since. I love not knowing what's coming in that door, then having to figure out how I can save a life, or what can I do to make this person better. It's like a hundred new puzzles that I have to solve every day.

I separate home and job completely. When I go home, I leave the ER at the hospital. It took me a few years, but I've learned how to block out everything that happens during my shift. If I took home some of the things I see at work, I'd be crazy as hell. I wouldn't be able to sleep. I'll tell you the truth—if I haven't seen it by now, I really don't *want* to see it.

Every day I see somebody die from a stabbing or a gunshot, or a motorcycle wreck. I used to talk about it with my fiancé, but he got tired of hearing it. Now people think I'm hard because almost nothing bothers me. That doesn't extend to my patients—they don't ever see the hard side of me unless they act like gutter trash.

The only things that bother me now are the dead babies or the sick children. On that, I cry more than the parents do. I've got five grandchildren and it just tears out my heart when those poor little children come into our ER.

It's been a full moon for the last two nights and it is sheer hell in that ER. That old full moon always makes the psych patients go real crazy and the traumas rise. When I look up and see that moon, I think, *Uh huh here we go. Roll up them sleeves.*

My first ER was in a poor black neighborhood. That was back when the police brought the dead bodies into the hospital to be pronounced. On my first day, I was told to go out to the ambulance and help bring in a girl who'd had her head chopped off with a machete by her boyfriend. That was my initiation.

I came into that same ER one morning not too long after that, and there was this young girl sitting outside on the waiting bench crying. All the other nurses weren't paying her any attention, so I just had to go see if I could help her. The other nurses warned me, saying, "Gloria, don't you go out there. Don't you do it, girl. You're new in this ER and you don't know anything about that thing out there."

I was shocked, so I said, "You're all so cold calling that poor girl a 'thing' like she's some kind of animal." I decided to show that girl some kindness, so I walked up on her and started talking to her for a few minutes to see what the trouble was, and just like that, *(she snaps her fingers)* she turned into something else, something not human. You'd have thought she was Satan himself. Oh my God, she was screaming and biting and cussing. It was so bad I thought I was going to faint.

I have learned not to trust what people tell me when they come into the ER. Like the night we had a young boy come in just as calm as a summer pond, even though he'd been shot through the stomach. He said he'd been walking down the street when someone shot him.

We were in the middle of treating him, when all of a sudden the police were on top of us. It turns out this boy had shot his father to death, but before the father died, he shot his son. After that I have never believed anything anybody tells me when they come in.

As far as the police go, I don't have any problems with them in my ER, at least not yet. They do their job, and if they're in our way I just say, "Look, it's your time to step out. This is *my* place. I don't come to your jail, getting in your way."

Another time a man came in complaining that it hurt him to sit down. The way he described it to me, it sounded like hemorrhoids, but when the doctor came to see him, he changed his story and said that he'd gone out drinking with his buddies and passed out and when he came to, his rectum was sore. The doctor did an exam and didn't find anything, but the man insisted something was there. He then changed his story again, and said that while he was working in his shop, he sat down on something hard, but didn't know what it was.

We sent him to be x-rayed and when it came back, we were standing around the x-ray box with our jaws hanging down. That man had a big old screwdriver stuck a foot up his rectum. We gave him a mess of muscle relaxants and managed to get it out in the ER.

Of course, the man didn't want us to tell his wife, but oh, I wanted so bad to say to that woman, "Girl, you need to quit him because that man is a total freak!"

The nurse working with me said, "Gloria, you're going to lose your job if you do that." But I was almost willing to take that chance.

That x-ray is still hanging in our ER. We have a collection of them— some with Coca-Cola bottles, light bulbs, rodents, vegetables, dildos, snakes—you name it, and I've seen it up there.

But you know, when you work ER, it messes with your head. We don't deal with the normal side of life. It's hard to think of anything good when you work the ER. You always think the worst. For instance, my son and his wife call me every day. Well, I hadn't heard from them for a whole day, so I called them, but nobody answered. I asked a friend who lives out that way to drive by, and she said both cars were in the driveway, all the lights were on, and there was mail in the mailbox.

Well, I just knew they were dead. I was sure they were in the house shot to death or cut up or something. I got so nervous, I called my daughter-in-law's mother, who finally told me they'd gone out of town.

It's so bad, I don't even allow my grandkids to play with balloons. I go to a kid's party and I take down all the balloons. People think I'm crazy, but I just tell them that I've seen too many kids come in brain dead or dead from balloons that got stuck in their airway.

The patients threaten us all the time, but who really pays attention to that? Patients and their family members, black and white, have hit me. We also have a lot of gang types coming in after gang wars. I recall one night looking out toward the triage nurse and I saw these three young black men coming through the door looking like they had something bad on their minds. My mind clicked and I thought to myself, *Oh-oh, better get out of the way!* so I started running.

The triage nurse saw the look on my face and she started running too, and pretty soon the whole staff was running. It turned out that nothing happened, but the look on those boys' faces was mean. I just figured they were coming in looking to kill the victim we'd just saved.

Then there was this lady who came in one night to see her son who'd been shot out on the street. I was the one who told her that her son was dead. She just looked at me and said, "This is my third son that got shot and died on the street."

My minister's wife was one of the ER doctors working that night, so I got her to come over and comfort that woman. What can you say to a mother who lost three sons to guns?

There are a lot of crazies out there now. They come in all shapes, colors and sizes. I'll never forget this little ten-year-old boy who came from California to live with his grandparents on account of him being too much to handle for his drugged out parents.

The boy was so bad, that during the flight out from California, they had to land the plane and put him into security. The grandfather had to drive to whatever state it was they let him out in and get him.

Two days later, the boy pushed the grandmother down the stairs and the grandfather called the police because he was afraid of the boy. The police couldn't do anything with him because of his age and all, so they brought him to the hospital in leather restraints.

That child called me every name under the sun, including names that even *I* hadn't heard before—that's how much cursing he was doing. The police put him in the psych ward until they could figure out what to do with him. Ten years old, can you imagine?

I had a nice-looking young brother come in one night who'd been shot through the abdomen out on the streets. He drove himself to another hospital and had to wait to be seen. Once they saw him they held him too long before transferring him to us. But still, he came in alert and oriented. I remember him holding onto my arm and saying, "Ma'am, am I gonna live?"

I told him, "Oh sweetheart you're going to live, I promise. You're going to be okay. Let's just see what the doctors say." I stuck with him right up until they came to take him to surgery. He died on the table and I felt so bad because I'd promised him he was going to be okay.

ER isn't all terrible, though. Some funny things happen too. Like the seven-year-old boy who came in with a sprained wrist. It was during a time when I was wearing my hair a purple color. This little boy kept on looking at me funny.

Finally he calls me over, "Hey you!" he says, looking real puzzled. "Why you got that Crayola head?"

Everybody laughed for weeks over that one. I finally had to change the color of my hair because everybody started calling me Crayola.

There was a drunk who came in all the time who had bad seizures that would almost kill him. One day I said, "Melvin, if you clean up, I'll marry you."

Well, if that man didn't go and get sober. Then he started coming to see me every day. He even brought his mother to meet me and told everybody I was going to be his wife. The staff would see him coming and they'd shout, "Hey Gloria, your fiancé is coming to see you."

After about three months, he came in having seizures because he'd started drinking again. All I could think was, *Thank you Jesus for getting me out of that mess.* Then I went in and told him, "Melvin, I'm sorry, but it's over between us."

I learned my lesson though—I'll never tell anybody anything like that again.

I never allow the patient's family to come into the rooms—I think it's completely unprofessional. They're always in the way, and that gets on my nerves, especially when you find them trying to see what's going on down the hallway with somebody that isn't any of their business. Then there are the ones who hit the floor the minute they see a needle, and suddenly you have two patients instead of one.

We have lots of people come in with cockroaches in their ears. Those patients are always jumping around all over the place when they first come in because they're going crazy with the noise the bugs make up against their eardrums trying to get out. We have to drop oil or liquid lidocaine into their ears to drown the roaches.

I'm not sure why, but we get lots of abortion patients in the summer. I remember back in the eighties we had a lot of teenaged girls come in hemorrhaging and septic because they'd tried to give themselves abortions. They would take a coat hanger and use the point to puncture the water bag and then they'd end up with a massive infection. I can't even tell you how many of those young girls died of sepsis.

Then there's all that white light stuff. I've had plenty of patients tell me about the white light they see when they've come up to death's door. They all say the same thing—they can see us all around working on them, but they want to go to that white light because it's so joyful.

Girl, I am telling you right now, if that light comes my way, and it's as full of joy as everybody says, nothing and nobody is going to be pulling me back, because I'll be gone.

NANCY ISSING
St. Vincent's Hospital, ER nurse
Lifelong New York City resident

"I have always wanted to be a nurse with the exception of a brief time in the fourth and fifth grades when I wanted to be a flight attendant or a nun.

"I was born in St. Vincent's Hospital. In high school I was a candy striper at St. Vincent's. Now I work full time at St. Vincent's and live less than a five-minute cab ride away.

"I will warn you right now that my emotions are still very much at the surface around this, and I still become tearful at times just thinking about it."

September 11, 2001
New York City

It was my first day off after working three 8 a.m. to 8 p.m. shifts in a row, so I was really looking forward to spending that first day doing absolutely nothing.

I was asleep when the phone rang about nine a.m. It was my brother calling to tell us to turn on the TV and that a small plane had crashed into the World Trade Center. As soon as I saw the tower with all that smoke billowing out, I thought, *Oh my God, I'll bet we're probably going to get a couple of patients from that.*

Obviously I had no idea what the magnitude of the disaster was at that point. I figured St. Vincent's might receive a few burn patients—maybe ten or twenty at most. I called the charge nurse, but the clerk didn't even put me through. She just said, "Come in now! We need you."

I dressed in front of the TV in the bedroom listening to a reporter talk about what type of plane was involved in the accident when, through the bedroom window, I heard this horrible, noise like, '*Whrroooomm!*' A split second later I saw the image of a jet going into the second tower on the TV.

I was shocked, unable to think properly. Even though the reporters were saying that there was a problem with air control at one of the airports, I started to get the feeling that maybe it was a terrorist attack. A few minutes later, my husband and I left the apartment together. As we went our separate ways, I looked over my shoulder at him, and for a split second I wondered if I was ever going to see him again.

Caught up in the urgency of getting to work, I was frustrated that I couldn't find a cab, and the buses were really slow. I finally caught a bus, but it felt like it was taking forever to get to St. Vincent's. At every intersection everyone would look south toward the towers, and every time I saw them burning, the need to get to work became all that more pressing.

I finally got off the bus and ran the rest of the way. All along the streets people were gathered around cars that had their radios on, blasting reports of what was happening.

Approaching the corner where I'd no longer be able to see the buildings, I slowed and took a last long look at the towers. Even now, I find myself still looking for them in that empty space in the sky where my eyes were used to finding them.

9:30 a.m.
I walked into St. Vincent's ER, amazed at how quickly they'd mobilized people and supplies. They'd already set up police barricades, and had stretchers lined up in the front of the building.

At that point we hadn't received any patients, but I was running over in my mind everything we'd have to do. I was there in 1993 when the World Trade Center was bombed, so I was gearing up to disaster mode, thinking in terms of burns and blast injuries and how we'd treat them.

Suzanne Pugh, my nurse manager, told me I was to be captain of Unit Five, which is the critical care area. My stomach flipped with apprehension until I spoke with the doctor who was going to be working with me and we outlined what we were going to do. I broke the room down into certain areas for the different types of patients we'd see. I had just enough time to go over the supplies, when the first survivors hit the door.

From that point of time until the patients stopped coming in is a big blur. Once the patients started coming in, I was completely focused on what I was doing: get a deep intravenous line in, get an airway in, and get them upstairs to the medical intensive care unit. Most of the patients I saw were badly burned, crushed, or in cardiac arrest.

I remember certain small pieces in great detail, such as the smell of the smoke that arrived with the first patients—like burning rubber-covered wires, and the smell of jet fuel on the burn survivors. After the buildings collapsed, everyone who came in was covered with those smells, and fine gray soot.

For months afterward, every rescue worker who came in smelled of that smoke. Even at home I would have to close all the windows and turn on the AC just to lessen the smell a little. It was December before the fire stopped burning and the smell finally faded.

All survivors had to have a bronchoscopy of their throat and vocal chords to see if they had any inflammation or burns—in case they needed an airway. There were a lot of anesthesiologists there, all of them ready to jump down everybody's throat—literally.

Where I was working was like a cocoon—there were no windows, no TV and no radio, so we were pretty isolated. Even if we'd had a TV or radio, there was no way we could have stopped what we were doing long enough to pay attention. Any information we got about what was going on outside came from the paramedics and the EMTs who brought the patients to us from Ground Zero.

Those first survivors were very badly burned. Unfortunately, most of them were conscious. There was one woman in particular who had burns over ninety percent of her body. I remember looking into her eyes and seeing a combination of terror and blankness. I don't know how to describe that look, but it really affected me. I remember taking her shoe off and the top of her foot where her shoe had been wasn't burned, but all the rest of her was. I don't know why I remember that so clearly, but I do. It was another one of those small detail things that stuck in my mind.

Someone else was trying to intubate her and someone else was getting a deep line into her and at the same time a couple of surgeons were trying to debride her burns and do wound care.

I realized that she wasn't sedated enough. They'd given her a strong sedative but it wasn't enough for her, not with the extent of those burns. She sat up at one point and stared at me with her eyes bugging out of her head, trying to scream—but she couldn't because of the breathing tube.

I got panicky then, feeling like I was part of a torture team. I rapidly infused Propofol, a drug used as a general anesthetic, into her IV. I didn't care what it did to her blood pressure—if it dropped it out, we'd deal with it later. I just wanted her to be unconscious. I wanted so much to take…to take away— (long pause)—to take all that horribleness away from her.

I was told she died, but I remembered her name because I kept track of everyone I gave narcotics to. Three weeks ago there was a news feature about a woman who'd been released from NY Cornell Burn Center. Of course her face had been badly burned, but when they said her name, I realized it was that woman, and I was so happy to see she was alive.

That day, I mostly remember their faces and that shocked expression that really wasn't any expression at all. I don't know what those patients were thinking, or even if they were thinking. I wasn't talking to them because I was in the I-need-to-take-care-of-this-immediately nurse mode—IV and airway, IV and airway.

We weren't doing bloods or EKGs or anything like that. Everything was geared toward stabilizing them, and then clearing them out of the ER as quickly as possible to make room for the other victims coming in.

I couldn't say at what point in the day I grasped the magnitude of what had happened, but I remember being afraid that we weren't going to be able to handle all of them, even though there were tons of staff.

A policeman told us at one point that they weren't allowing any rescue workers into that immediate area because the buildings were too unstable and they looked like they were going to fall. I had this terrible thought that there might be patients who needed to get to us, but the workers couldn't get to them.

We got a lot of people who had been crushed in the rubble. There was another rescue worker who—(long pause). You know, I almost don't want to talk about this man, because I don't want his family to know how badly his body was destroyed. When he first came in, I thought he was an old man, his hair was so gray from that soot, but as I looked at his face, I realized he was very young, maybe in his twenties. I think he'd been crushed in the rubble, or by something, I don't know, but by the time he got to us, he was dead. I guess the force of one of the explosions or whatever it was that fell on him, caused an implosion inside his body.

Still, we worked on him for a while and I remember looking down and seeing that his scrotum had been blown open and there was a part of it lying on his thigh. At first I thought it was his testicle attached to the spermatic chord, but while they were bagging him, it started to blow up and I realized it was his intestines.

When I saw that, I said, "We aren't going to get this man back. We need to stop." But, of course, we didn't stop. Even though I knew he was dead, we quickly got him into the trauma room to crack his chest.

His arm was hanging out over the side of the stretcher, and as they were pulling him in, way too fast, his arm hit the side of the cart. I screamed out loud, "Watch his arm!" I was so horrified that his arm would get hurt. It was crazy. His body was totally blasted to pieces and I was concerned about his arm.

I know it was an odd thing to remember, but I still see that boy's arm and it's very upsetting to me. It was such an incongruous thing to say, because at that point, it didn't really matter what— (long pause—tape turned off).

I was on vacation in St. Lucia that December and I was lying on the beach in this absolute paradise, looking at the water without a care in the world, thinking how beautiful it was, and BOOM—the image of that boy's arm just came right into my mind.

I remember being startled by it and thinking, *Whoa! Where did that come from?* It was so disturbing. You'd think other things would be worse, but that bothered me terribly.

Looking back on it now, I think the paramedics and EMTs were so desperate to do their job to help save people that perhaps they imagined they felt a pulse and they'd pick people up and bring them in even though they were actually dead. There weren't too many like that, thank God.

After the buildings collapsed, we didn't get many more patients. That was the frustrating part. A few times I went out to the ambulance dock on Seventh Avenue and stood there saying, "Come on! Let's go! Where are the patients? Why aren't they bringing us patients?" The quiet was almost enough to make us want to go down there and get the patients ourselves. We didn't understand then that there wouldn't be many more coming in.

My adrenaline level was still up, but I had this sick sort of mental and physical exhaustion. I didn't feel like sitting down, but on the other hand, I knew that my adrenaline level had been sustained for too long.

I restocked everything while I was still waiting for more patients. I was thinking, *Okay, they can't get to the patients now, but once they get in there, that's when we're really going to start seeing them.* I was thinking of how, when volcanoes erupt or there are earthquakes, rescue workers are able to dig people out sometimes days and weeks afterwards.

I was so hopeful. Even if I had seen the TV coverage, I still would have been hopeful. Being a nurse, I didn't know any of the mechanics of engineering or how compressed the floors were.

When Suzanne said to go home and she'd see me the next day, I was shocked. I thought she was crazy. I said, "What do you mean go home? I'm not going home! How can I go home now?"

But then the nightshift showed up and everyone was just sitting around waiting. I thought then that maybe Suzanne was right and I should get some rest because the next day was going to be really busy when they started pulling out the survivors.

About a block from the hospital I realized there was no traffic. It felt like a ghost town. No cars. No buses. The stores were all closed. It was creepy. Silent. At every intersection were police barricades with National Guardsmen and state troopers.

I felt heavy and alone because I realized that no one I was passing in the street could possibly imagine what I'd seen and done that day. I felt disconnected from everyone. I don't know why the staff didn't sit down and talk about their feelings with each other. We'd say how horrible it was, and that we couldn't believe it was happening, but nobody talked about how it was affecting them personally. I wish we'd done that. It might have helped a little.

When I got home, I turned on the TV and saw all the images for the first time. It didn't seem real. That was when I realized there would be no more survivors.

I don't remember when I first cried—it might have been in the shower that night, but I'm not sure. I might have talked about it with my husband, but not in any great detail. I don't remember if I slept or not.

September 12, 2001

The only patients we got were firemen, policemen and National Guardsmen coming in with lacerations, extremity injuries, fractures, eye injuries, and smoke inhalation problems.

We got a big golden retriever rescue dog named Bear who was dehydrated and had a large laceration of his thigh. Our doctor sutured him back up, we ran in some IV fluids, he rested for a while, and was discharged just like a regular patient.

Later in the day, a policeman came in who was so distraught he had to be sedated. I don't remember what his injury was, but his level of emotional distress was more than I'd seen that day. When we talked to his colleagues they said he'd lost his partner of many years and they figured he was dead. It turned out his partner was his K9 cop dog.

September 14, 2001

I was walking down the street and saw the lines of people waiting to donate blood. I realized then how incredibly lucky I was that I was a nurse and had been given the opportunity to help. I felt sorry for the people who weren't able to help, yet wanted to.

September 15, 2001

A group of us went down to Ground Zero triage center after work because they were asking for relief nurses and supplies. After dropping off the supplies, I went to the actual site.

People were walking around in protective gear suits that I'd never seen before except in the movies—they looked like spacemen. The smoke was very heavy and our eyes were burning, but I felt like I was on a movie set in a theme park like at MGM studios. I expected someone to jump out and yell, 'Action!'

My husband didn't understand how I could watch the tributes on TV, but I felt if I didn't listen to these people's stories, I was dishonoring them or turning my back on who they were and letting them down.

Recently a young broker who had been working in the World Trade Center that day and who'd been badly burned came back to visit us. He still had the compression bandages on his arms and hands, but his eyebrows were growing back in. His face was very scarred, but he looked beautiful to me.

I'm sure this has affected and changed my life on some level, but I'm not really sure how. I know I want to hug my children more. I feel as though I'm still in—

(pause)—still in the process of—(long pause—tape turned off).

Nurses from around the country and around the world were so wonderful in reaching out to us. There was such an outpouring of love and support. They sent telegrams, letters, and emails from as far away as Australia, offering support and praise.

After a while I felt embarrassed by all of the gratitude. It isn't as if we did anything more than other nurses would do in any other ER in the country. We didn't do anything more than we do every day, except on a much grander scale. Sometimes I want to say, "Oh please, stop the hero stuff!"

If the same thing happened again tomorrow, I would still respond the same way—anybody would. I'm a nurse. It's what I do—it's my job.

JESSICA

"My love affair with ER nursing began while I was a successful architect making a large salary. One day, my three-month-old son became ill so I took him to my HMO ER. There, the doctor scolded me for being an hysterical, over-reactive parent and sent me home with Tylenol. My gut told me he was wrong, so instead of going home, I drove to another ER. As I walked into the lobby, my son's heart and lungs stopped working.

"I ran to the first nurse I saw, begging her to save him. She took him from me and disappeared behind the double doors to the trauma room. After supplying the triage nurse with as much information as I could, I was led to the meditation room where a video had been left running about LifeFlight nurses.

"While they worked to keep my only child alive, I sat there watching that video and thinking that if my baby survived, I would dedicate my life to saving other people. My son made it through, so six months later, I closed up my practice and went to nursing school.

"I also volunteered in the local ER, and one night a young mom came running in and handed me this limp, hypoxic baby and started screaming to save her child. I took one look at that baby and got such a rush of adrenaline that I knew ER was the only place for me.

> *"I have worked ER for fifteen years, and although I graduated from law school and now plan to specialize in Constitutional and bioethics law, I won't stop working as an ER nurse completely—it's a part of the fabric of my life.*
>
> *"The best thing I've learned working in ER is that no matter what goes wrong in my life, I know how to keep it together. Like most nurses, I am a survivor."*

In the ER where I work, my nickname is Code Blue, because every time I'm on, we get one code after the other. I'm not complaining. There's nothing I like better than to be in the middle of adrenaline-charged chaos, putting it right.

I've slipped my hand inside a person's chest and actually held the heart. I've pulled newborns out of women with as much ease as I've put bodies into body bags—known as 'the final vinyl' and zipped them up.

This story might provide an incentive for people to carry Do Not Resuscitate orders with them at all times, or perhaps have it tattooed on their chests. This story also confirms all those buried alive horror stories you heard at summer camp—the ones that fueled your nightmares for years until you grew up and dismissed them as fiction. I now offer proof positive that they weren't fiction at all.

We got a radio call on an eighty-eight year old guy who collapsed at his best friend's funeral. The paramedics, transmitting from the gravesite, informed us that the old man was in ventricular fibrillation. They'd defibrillated him about six times and had maxed-out on all the pre-hospital medications. From this information, we knew that this scenario was not going to have a happy ending.

It was one of our ER policies that if the patient coming in was over the age of fifty and had been down for more than ten minutes, we were to automatically put the shroud bag down on the gurney so we can just zip them up if and when they didn't make it.

By the time the old gentleman got to us, he was dusky, his pupils were dilated and non-reactive, he wasn't breathing, and his rhythm had deteriorated to electrical-mechanical dissociation, which meant that his heart wasn't beating. For the next forty-five minutes we worked our butts off to get his heart going again, and failed. Finally, the physician called off the code and let him go.

I cleaned him up and put a fresh sheet over the body, and then I went to inform the family of his passing. The wife came back first and there followed such a tender, tearful farewell scene, we were all sobbing right along with her. More tears were shed when the kids and the grandkids came in. By the time it was over, I was truly sorry we hadn't saved the man—he sounded like a wonderful old soul.

However, life does go on, and after everyone left the room, I got back to the business of getting him down to cold storage because there was another code coming in and we needed the bed. I removed the monitor leads, tied on the toe tag and began zipping up the final vinyl. That was when I heard the soft, eerie sound.

"Eeeeeemmm."

I looked around the room, searching for the source of the noise. It had to be some electrical blip with the overhead lights, I thought, and resumed zipping until I again heard the strange sound.

I stopped zipping and put my ear next to the old man's mouth and listened—nothing. I felt for a carotid pulse—again, nothing.

"It's only a reflex," I said aloud. "Probably air escaping from his stomach."

The zipper was about nipple level when I thought I saw his chest move. I shook my head and dismissed the thought, chalking it up to a momentary hallucination. Unfortunately, just as I got the zipper past his nose, I couldn't ignore the fact his eyes fluttered open and he blinked.

I unzipped the bag and put my ear to the end of his endotracheal tube. Goosebumps broke out all up and down my arms at the sound of faint respirations. I placed the pulse oximeter on his finger, and sure enough, he had an oxygen saturation of eighty-six percent. I quickly hooked him back up to the cardiac monitor and right there on the screen was a limping rhythm, but a rhythm all the same. His blood pressure proved to be better than mine.

Even then I thought to myself, *Jess, just zip up the damned bag. He's eighty-eight and his brain is totally fried. Zip up the bag and don't say a word to anybody about this. No one ever has to know.*

But, I was raised Catholic, and all those stories about burning in Hell for eternity came to mind, so I started yelling for help, giving up any hope I may have had of working for Dr. Kevorkian.

The doctor showed up first and asked what the hell I was yelling about, so I told her to check the monitors. She took one look, went pale and said, "Jess, just zip up the bag and take him to the morgue. We'll swear we never saw it."

I told her I couldn't do it, and that she would have to be the one to take him to cold storage. Unfortunately, she was raised Catholic too, so neither one of us could zip up the bag.

I went to the waiting room praying to God that the family would have already gone home, but no such luck. They were all still there, assembled in a prayer group, praying for Gramp's dearly, but not quite departed, soul.

I approached them wondering how many lawsuits were going to be filed as a result of this fiasco. Praying they had a sense of humor, I smiled and said, "I have some good news. It seems Gramps was only kidding. He's been resurrected and is now alive." What I neglected to add was that he was alive *in body only*, and that his mind had vacated the premises hours ago.

The family came in, and at the sight of this old guy with his eyes open, all pinked up and breathing, pandemonium broke out. The wife fainted from the strain of the whole experience, the children were in shock, and the grandkids were confused. Everyone was asking questions none of us could answer.

The old man died the next day and stayed dead long enough for ICU to get the final vinyl zipped and down to cold storage, thank God.

From that time on, whenever a patient dies after we've coded him, we look at each other and whisper, "Just zip up the bag!"

APRIL

"When I was a paramedic, stabilizing, loading up and hitting the road wasn't enough. I wanted to have more to do with what took place after we scraped up the pieces. I chose to be a nurse because it seemed to be the next logical step. Sometimes, when I can't sleep at night after seeing what I see in the ER, I wonder if I made the right decision.

"More and more I see my colleagues turn off their compassion and empathy because they're overwhelmed. It makes me sick the way healthcare has been turned into one big corporate greed machine. It's for that reason that there isn't much caring in healthcare anymore."

The five-year-old girl in the blue gingham dress and black patent leather shoes wears that telltale hangdog look kids get when they've been abused. It's something that hides behind the eyes, as if the soul inside is looking out at you through a haze of smoke. The pain is hidden, but screaming in your face at the same time. I see it the second I walk into the treatment room, and my heart drops to my knees. The child's name is Rose and she is delicate and small and beautiful.

I look at the chart to hide my expression and read the vague complaint given by the mother. *"Mother states her daughter has leg sores."*

Mom is well dressed and appears fairly normal by ER standards. By that I mean there aren't any track marks on her arms, she's clean and doesn't reek of alcohol, urine, or worse.

I make the mistake of touching the child's hand. Instantly Rose pulls away and hides in the folds of her mother's sweater. I give mom a sympathetic look and hand her a pediatric hospital gown with pink teddy bears in the design. I ask her to undress her daughter, and tell her I'll be right back. I then go to the nurses' station to gather the child abuse forms I know I'll eventually need.

I am walking across the ER lobby when I see Dr. A arrive. Dismayed, I clench my jaw. Dr. A is a burned out ER doc who, as far as I know, has never shown one iota of compassion or kindness toward anyone.

Rose's mother begins to explain the moment I open the treatment room door. "I've been divorced from Rose's father for about two years," she says, never once looking me in the eye. "He has her on the weekends."

There is silence while she brushes a few wispy strands of Rose's thin, dark hair behind the girl's ears. "When he brought her back a few weeks ago, I noticed these red marks on her—" Her voice falls to a whisper and goes silent. She lifts the hospital gown and points to the child's genitalia.

I already know what I'm going to see, so I don't visibly react, but my throat gets tight. I have seen these injuries so many times over the years that I'm amazed it still affects me this way. The raw red flesh of her labia matches the collection of bruises and welts that line her inner thighs.

"At first I thought she'd been sliding down the banister in my husband's apartment building," the mother continues. "But this week, I thought I'd better come here and make sure that's what it is."

"What does Rose say about all this?" I ask, glancing at the child.

"She doesn't. When I ask her how she got hurt, she pretends not to understand."

I stare at the mother. It isn't rocket science to figure out what is going on, and for the hundredth time I'm at a loss to understand mothers who live in that vast, numbing state of Denial.

I nod and make a few notations on the anatomical drawings to show exactly where the bruises, welts, and outer labial tears that I can see, are located. Distracting the girl with a balloon, I take an earprobe temperature, count her respirations and pulse, note them on the chart, and tell Mom I'll be back with the doctor in a moment.

All the way to the charting desk, I feel like I'm being violated by a bunch of disorderly emotions: anger, sadness, pity, fear, and worst of all, the desire to turn it off and fall into the comfortable arms of apathy.

Dr. A does a cursory visual exam of the child's injuries without uttering one word to mother or child. He exits the room with a mumbled instruction to put ointment on the worst of the wounds and then heads for the clerk's desk to prepare discharge papers. I follow him down the hall, my mouth flapping. "Hey, wait! Aren't you going to do a vaginal exam? This child has been sexually molested."

He pulls the child abuse forms out of the chart and shoves them at me. "What the hell are you trying to do?"

"We need the child abuse report forms filled out," I reply. "CPS requires them before they'll investigate a case."

He looks me straight in the eye and leans so close, I can smell the coffee on his breath. "This case is a can of worms. Refer her to a private pediatrician. I don't intend on spending my days off testifying in a courtroom."

I stare at him. "That little girl needs your protection. The mother needs a doctor to verify that there's evidence of sexual abuse."

"I'm not signing them," he says and walks away.

"Fine," I say. "I'll sign them myself."

And I do. I fill out the abuse forms then call Child Protective Services. As I punch in the numbers, it dawns on me that it's a sad state of affairs that I have memorized the number from using it so much.

A husky female voice answers with an irritated sigh. I explain who I am and tell her about Rose.

In return, she asks for Rose's name, date of birth, description of injuries and the mental state of both the mother and child. Then she asks if the doctor has filled out and signed the form yet.

"No, because he doesn't want to be called into court to testify. I've filled them out and signed the form as an RN. That's legal in this state."

"Oh," she says and then there's this long pause during which I pray she won't hang up. "Well, in that case, there's nothing CPS can do for you."

"I'm not asking that you do something for me," I say, my voice turning snarky. "I need you to do something for this five-year-old child who is being sexually abused by her father on a weekly basis."

To my horrified amazement, the woman laughs. "If the doctor won't sign the forms stating that there is physical evidence of sexual abuse, we can't do anything for the child, so put away your sad violin and find a doctor who *will*." She hangs up without a goodbye.

I sit listening to the dial tone, choking on the lump of frustration and anger that has become part of my daily diet and return to Rose and her mom.

Rose is curled up on mom's lap sucking her thumb. I sit down, sigh, and in one long, run-together sentence, tell mom the doctor blew them off because he's an inhuman bastard, and she can't depend on CPS because they basically don't care, and that what she really needs to do is bring Rose to a private pediatrician, and then hire an attorney, and under no uncertain circumstances should she let the child return to her father until the authorities have looked into the matter.

I give her a pediatric referral, dispense samples of antibiotic ointment and a hug for mom, and walk out feeling like I've stepped on a land mine. For the hundredth time I have been left with my ass hanging out to dry without the backing of the CPS or the doctor.

I turn the corner into the main receiving room and see a boy of maybe nine being wheeled in by an EMT and a cop. Trailing behind the gurney are two younger children, and the mother, who appears unsteady on her feet.

The boy's face is covered with blood; his expression is one of angry indignation. The other two children, a boy of maybe five and a girl about seven, are wearing the hangdog look.

The EMT hands me the 911 report. During a domestic violence scene the mother's boyfriend punched the boy and knocked him unconscious. One of the neighbors called the police and the boyfriend was hauled off to jail.

At the bottom of the report is a note signed by one of the paramedics. *Neighbors report that there have been repeated violent attacks on the three children by mother's boyfriend. Please call CPS for placement.*

I focus on the mother who is either drunk or stoned—probably both. She begins to spout off and it's clear that she's flipping out, not because her son has been hurt, but because her boyfriend is in jail. In fact, she's downright indignant and in the middle of the main room, stops to tell the cop what an asshole he is for arresting 'her man'.

I give in to the insanity. Tonight the blue light special is going to be abused kids and I will just have to deal with it.

I steel myself and quietly slip into the fray. I guide the three kids to the back treatment room. No one seems to notice our departure because mom is in center ring bellowing, playing it up for every bit of attention she can get.

I gather child abuse forms and settle in with the kids who, at first glance, all appear exhausted and undernourished. The injured boy, Dave, feigns indifference, an obvious front for his younger siblings who introduce themselves as Tiffany and Danny.

"Wow," I say as I examine Dave's injuries. "That must really hurt."

Dave shrugs and looks away. "Not really."

"Looks to me like that nose might even be broken." I apply a soft cold pack to the bridge of his nose. "Is this the first time this guy has ever hit you?"

"He hits us all the time," his sister pipes in at full volume. "But Dave gets it more than me or Danny because he's older."

"Shut up Tiffany," Dave says, disgusted and embarrassed at the same time.

Hands on hips, Tiffany strikes an indignant little sister pose. "Well he DOES, Davie, and you know it!"

"Yeah," says Danny putting in his two cents, "he hits us hard and straps us too!"

As if this were their cue, both Tiffany and Danny lift their tops. Under the grimy jerseys live a hundred bruises and purple strap marks of varying sizes and ages. Their bodies look like thin, white punching bags that have recorded every hit in purple, yellow, and blue.

I take a deep breath and sit on the exam stool so I can be eye level with them. "I see what you're showing me and I hear what you're telling me. I'm on your side. I'm not sure what I can do, but I'm going to try to help you."

All three children stare at me as if mesmerized, so I continue. "No one should ever hit you. It isn't right and you don't ever deserve to be hit—ever. Do you know that it's against the law to hit someone, especially children?"

Their eyes grow wide as saucers. Nobody so much as blinks.

"Jail sounds like a safe place for the person who hit you. You know, sort of like when they give you a time out in school for misbehaving?"

"I wish he would go to jail and stay there forever," Tiffany says in a low, sulky voice.

Danny punches the air and makes a noise that sounds disturbingly like a fist hitting flesh and says, "I wish he'd die."

Dave looks over the side of the gurney at the floor and mumbles something about blowing the son of a bitch away.

"Where's your father?" I ask, already thinking of ways to bypass CPS.

"He was a loser too," Dave says, not taking his eyes off the floor. "He left us before Danny was even born."

I put my arm around his shoulder and feel him melt under my touch. Tiffany and Danny immediately pull my free arm around their shoulders.

"Do you have any aunts and uncles," I ask.

They look uncertain, as if they aren't sure what an aunt or uncle is, so I clarify. "You know, like relatives other than your mom?"

"You mean, like Grandma?" Tiffany asks.

Relieved, I nod. "Where does your grandma live?"

"In M—," Dave says, then adds, "We don't see them very much because Butthead doesn't want us to go there, and he won't let them come to our house."

M— is ten miles away. I ask Dave for Grandma and Grandpa's last name and tell them I'm going to do everything I can to make sure they're safe for the night. What I don't say is that if I have to, I will try to arrange with CPS to take them home with me, even if I lose my job over it.

I leave them with toys and books and go in search of the mother. I find her talking on the phone to a bail bondsman, making arrangements to spring Butthead from jail.

"If I don't get him out of the hole tonight, he'll kill me," the mother tells me. I know from the way she's hyperventilating, she isn't kidding. I also know why she has a foot-stomping hissy fit when I tell her that the children will not be going home with her even if Butthead does get out of jail.

"Lady, if them kids aren't there when he gets home, he's gonna beat the shit outta *me!* The kids can take it better. They've got to go home with me, or I am one dead bitch." She says this without a hint of shame or remorse.

I have to restrain myself from giving my true thoughts a voice. Instead, I find the grandparents in the phone book and call them. I'm not surprised that they're extremely reluctant to get involved.

"We're old and both in poor health," Grandma says before I can even ask them to come in and take temporary guardianship of their grandchildren.

"We're already in bed," Grandpa adds from the extension phone. "I don't think it would be wise for us to come down there."

From where I'm standing, I see the mother charge through the main room. She tells the clerk she's going to the jailhouse but she'll be back in a half hour. I wave my arms to get the clerk's attention, silently mouthing 'no.' The clerk gives me a what-can-I-do shrug.

"I'm sorry, but you must come in tonight," I say to the grandparents. It is a command, not a request.

There is such a long silence on the other end of the line, that I think perhaps they have fallen asleep. I'm about to say something when Grandma sighs resignedly and says, "Oh all right!" and hangs up.

I run to the ambulance bay just in time to see the mother peeling out of the parking lot in the direction of the jail. When I return to the kids, Dr. A is examining Dave's nose and facial bones. Tiffany is chatting non-stop about Butthead and how he beats and straps them. The physician barely glances at the bruises and welts she and Danny display for him. I study his face, looking for a reaction. Nothing registers in those cold eyes and I know without asking that he will refuse to sign the CPS forms.

I am filling out the CPS paperwork when the grandparents shuffle in, he with a walker, and she with a cane. They appear to be in their mid-seventies and are indeed frail. I introduce myself and give them an impassioned pitch as to why they must take in their grandchildren, at least for the night.

"I don't think we should get involved," Grandpa says and looks at his wife for support. The wall of their reticence is so thick, I doubt they have heard one word I've said.

"This is the first man who has stuck by our daughter for more than a few months," Grandma says. "I know the man isn't perfect, but Barbara isn't an easy person to live with either. She's got her own ideas about what she wants to do with her life."

I show them to the treatment room, hoping the sight of the children's battered bodies will put a few cracks in the wall of their reluctance. The children are surprised and a little confused at the sight of these people who have never rescued them before. The grandparents seem embarrassed and perhaps, I hope, a little ashamed.

While they are all becoming reacquainted, I call CPS and leave a message. Fifteen minutes later I am called to the phone. When I put the receiver to my ear I can tell the caller is in a phone booth.

"Jesus H. Christ," the CPS field rep screams over the traffic noise. "Are you trying to tell me you got three kids who need placement *tonight?*"

"Yes," I say, and add, "Hopefully they can all go to one place. These kids are going to get the crap kicked out of them if they go back into that home. They're perfect for CPS foster care—they're eager to talk to any adult who will listen."

The CPS rep mutters something before the blast of a truck horn drowns her out. "Honey," she says finally, laughing bitterly, "I'm on a payphone with a station wagon full of kids who I don't know what the hell I'm gonna do with, so you better try to find something else for tonight. Send me the paper work, but right now I just don't have time for anything, especially three more damned kids to place. Call me back tomorrow."

I listen to the dial tone hoping she will suddenly come back on and say she's found a place for all of them, but I know she won't.

I walk back to the treatment room with a new sense of urgency and tell the grandparents that CPS doesn't have the resources right now, so they have no choice but to take the kids home with them.

The grandmother shakes her frail little white-haired head that I want to crush with my bare hands, and says, "No, I don't think so. We really don't want to interfere in our daughter's personal affairs."

I disassociate and look at the scene. I've got the littlest one hanging on for dear life to my one leg, and Tiffany hanging on to the other leg and Dave is pressed up under my arm. Their faces are turned up, their eyes pleading.

"Do you see these children?" I say to the grandmother who keeps her eyes glued to the floor. I bend down and force her to look at me. "These children are your own flesh and blood, and every one of them has been violently abused over and over again by the animal your daughter lives with, and she *lets him do it!*"

I realize I'm yelling, and lower my voice. "Are you telling me that you're going to let these children go back into that home tonight to be beaten, and possibly murdered?"

Grandma looks away and I move with the kids en masse in order to pick up eye contact again. "Your daughter is down at the jail as we speak posting bail for that monster. The second he gets home he's going to beat these kids again. Your daughter knows it, these kids know it, I know it, and I suspect you do too, so let's stop pretending it won't happen."

Grandma and Grandpa look at each other, and in that second, an entire conversation takes place between them.

"All right," Grandma says bitterly, as if she is agreeing to be shot at dawn. "We'll take them just for the one night, but after that, they have to—"

"Yippee!" yells Danny before she can finish. "We're going to Grandma's! Can we watch TV and have ice cream, Grandma?"

"Are you sure you can't take them for a few days?" I beg, "At least until CPS has a chance to evaluate the situation?" I know CPS will take at a month to get to the kids, but if I can get the children a least a week's reprieve from the violence, it will be better than no time at all.

Another look passes between the two grandparents. "We can't have them more than three or four days,"

Grandpa says. "My wife has arthritis and can't be running after kids. I don't like driving more than I can help it, and now I'll have to be driving them to and from school. It's not safe!"

I know enough not to push my luck and quickly begin packing the kids up before Grandma can change her mind and before Mom can get back with Butthead in tow for an old-fashioned domestic violence scene in the ER.

I give Dave's discharge instructions to Grandma and rush them out to the parking lot. Before they get into the car, I kiss each child and hold them close.

I will probably never know what ultimately happens to them, unless one of them comes in on a gurney beat up or dead. I want to tell them I am here for them and that if they need help, to come and see me. I open my mouth to say this, but all that comes out is a hollow whisper of despair.

LORRAINE ENSMINGER
Beth Israel Hospital, ER nurse manager
Lifelong New York City resident

"Some administrators would prefer that I stick exclusively to management, but I prefer to have a rapport with my staff, so I practice patient care whenever I get the chance. I'm not replacing anyone; I just need to keep in touch. It's easier for the nursing staff to relate to me and easier for me to understand what they're going through if I'm working alongside them. This makes me a more effective and compassionate leader.

"After all, I didn't take this job to be a pencil pusher; I took it because I wanted to practice nursing."

September 11, 2001
New York City

I arrived at my office before 7 a.m. and was greeted with the news that three staff members from the day and evening shifts had called in sick. About an hour and forty-five minutes into my shift, while I was still making calls to off-duty staff trying to get the sick calls covered, an elderly woman ran from the street into the emergency department screaming that a plane had just hit the World Trade Center.

Beth Israel does have a psychiatric service, so I automatically thought that the woman was having a psychotic episode and was in need of counseling. After all, if such a thing happened we would have heard about it.

In as understanding a tone as I could muster, I said, "Don't worry, that all happened back in nineteen forty-five when a plane hit the Empire State Building. You don't have to be afraid now. That's all over and done with."

But she insisted. "No! You don't understand! The World Trade Tower has been hit by a plane!" She was so adamant and so distraught, that I began to wonder if what she claimed was true. Before I could say anything more, a man dressed as a bicycle messenger ran up to the ER desk and yelled, "A small plane just flew into one of the World Trade Towers!"

I immediately went on alert. They couldn't both be mistaken, so I went to the ER desk and immediately called 911 dispatch. When the dispatcher picked up, I heard what sounded like the din of a crowded police station, with frantic voices in the background. I asked if there were any reports of an incident at the World Trade Center. The dispatcher's response was, "Yes, but I can't talk right now. Just tell me how many cases can you take."

Without hesitation, I answered, "We can take about a hundred."

"Fine," she said. "You've got it!"

As soon as I hung up, I realized that I'd just offered to take a hundred casualties in a 25-bed ER. I went to the patient waiting area to see how many people we had waiting to be seen. Glancing at the TV, I saw that the

North Tower was enveloped in smoke. It was like something out of a Bruce Willis movie, only this was reality.

I assessed the four waiting patients, and, seeing that they were minor complaints, asked if they could return another time or follow up with their family doctor. They all readily complied. One of them said, "We know you're about to be very busy."

With that, something clicked and I switched into disaster mode. We had to open up space for what was going to be a Code Orange—our name for an external disaster.

9:05 a.m.

We heard an announcement boom from the TV that another plane had hit the second tower. My staff and I looked at each other and my blood ran cold. These could not be two coincidental plane accidents—they had to be deliberate. Were we at war?

I needed to get a hold of administration, but every extension I dialed just rang until the out-of-office message came on. I called the Director of Nursing's office and her administrative secretary informed me that all administrators were attending a high level meeting at corporate headquarters up town.

"Then who's in charge?" I asked.

"I guess you are," she replied.

9:15 a.m.

The ER staff and I emptied out the pediatric area, the Fast Track, and the lobby and turned them into trauma treatment areas. The ER waiting room became a respiratory treatment area for smoke inhalation patients.

We focused on what sort of cases we would most likely see—trauma, respiratory, burns, and eye injuries. On a normal day, EMS would triage those cases to centers that specialized in the care they required, but this was not a normal day, and our trauma II level designation was irrelevant.

Transport went unit to unit rounding up every available stretcher and wheelchair they could find. On a good day, I couldn't find a stretcher to save my life; that day, they were coming out of the woodwork and not one wheelchair was missing a footrest.

Strangely enough, it was beautiful weather that day, so triage was set up outside the ER entrance. With the help of the NYPD and hospital security, we closed off Sixteenth Street and private vehicles were towed away to make room for the reception area.

9:45 a.m.

I used an outside line to call Administration again, and this time got a recorded message saying, "We are unable to connect this call because of a tornado in your area." I wasn't surprised that the phone company didn't have a message saying, "We are unable to connect this call because of terrorist activity in your area."

We continued in disaster mode, hanging IVs and getting stretchers and equipment in place. Additional staff began showing up from all over the hospital campus. Assignments were made and everyone had a role.

The first ambulances began showing up—cuts, bruises, shock, falls, chest pain. They were immediately triaged and brought in for treatment.

We heard that a highjacked airliner had just hit the Pentagon, and it dawned on me that the United States was in a fight for survival.

10:28 a.m.

We were treating a hundred plus patients who were spread out over the entire first floor, from the ER to the auditorium, when we heard a distant rumble. At the same time, a shout came over the EMS-hospital radio saying, "The North Tower has collapsed! Oh shit, the tower is down!"

I ran to the ER waiting room to look at the TV screen, and saw that it was true. All of those people were gone! I ran outside and informed my director. In disbelief she asked, "What do you mean collapsed?"

"There is no more World Trade Center," I said. "The towers are gone."

An acrid smell, like burnt electrical wiring, filled the air as a sprinkling of what looked like grey particles fell onto our faces, hair and clothing. We donned masks and protective eyewear to avoid getting it into our mouths and eyes.

The streets became eerily empty and quiet, and then suddenly, droves of people began rounding the corner of First Avenue onto 16th Street, and hurried towards the ER entrance. They converged on us, demanding surgical masks. We distributed what we could, and had to send someone to a hospital uptown for more.

11:00 a.m.

My thoughts turned to my husband who was an Emergency Service police officer stationed at 21st Street and Second Avenue, just blocks from Beth Israel. I knew that he and his colleagues would be at the scene. He'd worked the night before, but left me a message on our answering machine that he was returning to work at the towers.

Information from then on was hard to get. The phone lines were down all over New York, so communicating with other hospitals and authorities was next to impossible. Security began distributing satellite radios to those of us in charge.

The units continued to send down the extra staff who had been steadily arriving from their homes. Nurses and doctors from nearby hospitals and other medical centers in New York also came in to help. Dietary Services delivered cases of water, and food for staff, rescuers and patients. Civilians and shopkeepers also brought donations of food and clothing. Many begged to do something to help.

At this point we had triaged and were treating over 240 patients.

3:00 p.m.

Ambulances continued to arrive with survivors. Patients, staff and rescuers were now so covered in that grey dust, that we added gloves to our protective wear.

On a day where we had to be there for one another, it was significant that we couldn't distinguish what a person's race was. That day everyone was simply a human being. There was no such thing as different religions or different races. There was no contention between any two factions. That day, cops, firemen, nurses, physicians, paramedics, and civilians all played a role in rescuing and supporting one another. All the petty gripes that were usually such a big deal didn't matter anymore. That day we weren't black, white, brown, or yellow—all of us were gray, and everyone got VIP treatment.

All three of the staff members who called in sick earlier showed up, along with nearly a hundred percent of my entire twenty-four hour complement of emergency room staff.

3:30 p.m.

The ER was full of patients, the civilians looking for loved ones, and the officials from government agencies who were conducting interviews and collecting data.

Two policemen were brought in together by ambulance. Their injuries were not life-threatening, but they needed to be admitted for observation. They were absolutely adamant about not being separated from each other, to the point of insisting that they be on stretchers side-by-side in the ER. They weren't talking much, but it was clear they'd been through something traumatic together.

This is behavior one doesn't normally see in NYC policemen. NYPD cops have a well-known reputation for being tough guys who have seen it all. That day, they experienced things they weren't prepared for in the police academy.

One of the paramedics who brought them in told us that the two officers were among the first cops to arrive at the towers after the planes hit. They'd witnessed people jumping out of the windows. As the first tower collapsed, one of them was running to find shelter from the falling debris, when a large piece of falling steel hit a woman running a few feet in front of him and cut her in half.

When his partner caught up with him, the two continued to look for people in the debris, pulling on arms and legs or anything they could see that looked human. Except, when they pulled at the limbs, the rest of the person wasn't attached.

We received three critical trauma cases. One gentleman had sustained injuries from being crushed in the stampede when the towers fell, another was a young man who had been hit by concrete and was temporarily unconscious. There was also an older gentleman who escaped from one of the higher floors in one of the towers and had sustained multiple blunt trauma injuries.

The majority of the people who came in had simple fractures, lacerations, corneal abrasions and respiratory difficulty from the inhalation of dust and smoke.

4:00 p.m.

The arrival of patients slowed down dramatically, and at this point we were treating mostly rescuers who suffered minor injuries. It was becoming evident that there would be few if any survivors.

Because of this lag, I had time to focus on the needs of the staff. I didn't want to focus on myself because I didn't want to confront the fear of what may have happened to my husband. Without phone lines I couldn't locate him, and we'd not spoken or seen each other since the day before when he left home for his night shift. Worrying about that would have made me feel vulnerable, which would have impeded the way I functioned. Instead I concentrated on organizing a place for my staff to sleep.

The bridges and tunnels leading in and out of New York City had been shut down, so at least for tonight, the hospital was home. With help, I made sure the staff had enough to eat, and clean scrubs for a change of clothes.

4:30 p.m.
Some members of my staff and I went outside to wait for more patients. While standing in front of the ambulance dock, I looked north toward First Avenue and saw two police officers completely covered in that gray dust, walking toward the hospital. All I could think was, *Oh God, not another injured cop,* but then one of them smiled and began waving, and I realized the cop was my husband. He'd come to let me know he was alive and not to worry. It was the shot of adrenaline I needed.

After a few minutes he had to leave with his partner to re-join the search for survivors. He told me many rescuers were missing as well.

We kissed and said, "See you later." No goodbyes—not that day.

5:00 p.m.
Phone lines were working sporadically. A 911 dispatcher called asking if we had at least two hundred body bags. It was expected that casualties would be high and more bags would be needed downtown. I passed the task onto the pathology team.

Evening and night staff continued to arrive. Many of them had walked miles to get to the hospital—some from as far as Brooklyn and the Bronx. One of my RNs had walked from his house in Brooklyn across the Brooklyn Bridge. He was soaked in sweat and was exhausted, but he was full of enthusiasm and ready to work all night.

Two other RNs had hitched a ride across the Queensboro Bridge on the back of a *Newsday* truck. It was a surprise to see a newspaper delivery truck pull up to the ambulance entrance. The driver exited the cab, opened the back gate of the truck and announced, "Special delivery!" Two of our nurses jumped out raring to go. It was the first time anyone smiled that day.

I have always had respect for my staff, but I was in awe of their dedication. The camaraderie was amazing, and all the personality clashes had disappeared. I saw a lot of compassion—nurses taking care of nurses—and I was proud to be working with them.

5:30 p.m.

There was an announcement that WTC Building Seven had collapsed and hundreds of rescuers were lost.

I was not the only nurse married to someone in public service. There was one who was married to a paramedic, another to a fireman, and two other nurses who were married to police officers. We shared a morbid bond of predicting if we were going to be widows by morning. In silence we prayed and hugged one another for support and comfort.

I waited as long as I could and finally called my husband's precinct. When someone answered, I said, "This is Lorraine Ensminger. My husband is Officer Vernon Ensminger. Has anyone seen him? Can you tell me if he's okay?"

At first the man on the other end said he didn't know, but then called out my husband's name. An eternity went by, and when the phone was picked up, I heard my husband's voice.

I felt like I'd won the lottery. Knowing that he was all right, I was able to focus again. I asked him to call our twelve-year-old son who was staying at a friend's house. His friend's mother had called to say that my son was glued to the TV and would not take off his backpack, change his clothes, or eat until he heard from his father.

He'd spoken to me, but insisted he needed to hear his father's voice to be sure I wasn't keeping anything from him.

I told my husband I loved him and that I would see him the next day. He said he'd call our son and then head back down to Ground Zero to help find more victims—eight of whom were his fellow Emergency Service Unit officers.

After I hung up, I realized that I'd spoken to my husband in whispers. I felt guilty that I'd found him, because I knew that the other nurses still had not made contact with their spouses, and I didn't want to hurt anyone's feelings.

6 p.m.

Triage was empty. We'd not received an ambulance in over an hour. The city was quiet—no traffic, few pedestrians. The only people we saw now were in search of their loved ones. They were beginning to come in with photographs and descriptions of those who were missing, asking, "Have you seen my mom?" or, "Have you seen this woman? She's my wife."

Unfortunately, most of the time our answer was in the negative.

All New York City emergency rooms had faxed patient lists to each other to help make it easier for staff to cross-reference so the missing might be located at other facilities. It was a daunting task going through hundreds of names. Only twice that entire night did we have the opportunity to tell someone their loved one was safe. One of them was admitted to our hospital, and the other, admitted to another New York facility.

Out of all that had happened that day, our inability to tell people we had their loved one, was the worst part. We are nurses—we're supposed to help people. They came in looking to us for answers and comfort, and we had little or none to give. How could lists of hundreds of names produce such few results? Were all of these people still trapped under the towers?

11:00 p.m.

Many people asked if they could put up photos and descriptions on the external walls of the ER and ambulance bay. Without hesitation, we told them they could and even placed easels outside with boards where they could write messages and contact information.

September 12, 2001
1:00 a.m.

Not a single ambulance had arrived in hours, so we brought the stretchers and wheelchairs back inside.

Two of our surgical residents left for Ground Zero in one of our ambulances, hoping to help and maybe find out what happened to another one of our ambulances that had gone to Ground Zero soon after the planes hit, but had not been seen or heard from since. Two of our paramedics were missing. We would later find out that they had perished.

3:00 a.m.

Looking pale and wiped out, the surgical residents returned. The ambulance's right rear window was shattered and the interior was covered in that gray dust, as were both residents.

We asked what happened, and they just shook their heads and said that there was no one left to save.

4:00 a.m.

We stood outside all night just in case we were needed. People were starting to line up at the blood bank around the corner from the ER.

A man dressed in shorts and T-shirt rode up on a bicycle. Obviously stressed, he handed us a list of almost four hundred names, saying that they were his employees and he needed to find them.

One of my nurses, God bless her, sat with him and went through every one of those four hundred names, cross-checking it with all the patient lists from all the other hospitals. She didn't find a single name.

The man got back on his bicycle, thanked us and began to ride away. We asked where he was going. He answered that he didn't know.

Days later we found out that the man was a co-owner and CEO of a large brokerage firm that was located in one of the towers above where the planes hit. That day he hadn't gone to work earlier because it was his child's first day in pre-school. As fate would have it, he was the sole survivor of his firm.

Next, a Japanese tour guide came in looking for any surviving members of a Japanese tour group of 19 people, all of whom had been on the roof of one of the towers at the time it was hit. We knew we wouldn't find any of them, but we looked anyway.

For the rest of the night we smoked cigarettes. Even the non-smokers joined in. We did a lot of reminiscing, and drank a lot of coffee. We felt like old people sitting on a porch on some macabre farm looking down those abandoned streets where there was no traffic, only that eerie silence.

9:00 a.m.

Fresh staff began to arrive. The blood bank now had a line of donors stretching around the block.

Still dressed in my scrubs, I started for home. It was so strange riding the subway and having strangers come up to me to say "Thank you for all you've done."

And all I could say was, "You're welcome." But as far as I was concerned, thanks were not necessary. I did my job. My reward was to see my kids and wait for my husband to come home.

November 22, 2014

When I think of the aftermath of September 11, the first thing that comes to mind was having to deal with what I called the 'ER Syndrome.'

We saw 241 patients within two hours on September 11. The patients we saw that day required a much higher level of emotional and physical care than our usual, everyday patients.

After such an emotionally draining event, the staff had to relearn how to go back to normal and care for the non-traumatic, everyday patients who came in with commonplace complaints such as sprained ankles and the common cold. We've had to remember that all our patients are important, and even though they aren't part of a disastrous event, they deserve the same amount of care.

The patients who came in regularly for dialysis had to be called and asked to return to resume treatment. One of the dialysis patients told us he hadn't come in because he thought we were too busy with 'real patients' to take care of him anymore.

Soon after September 11, we saw an increase in the number of patients with symptoms of depression coming in for mental health services, along with a corresponding increase in alcohol use and suicide attempts. These problems were not exclusive to civilians. Healthcare workers and rescuers also suffered from depression and an increase in alcohol abuse.

There were prayer services, candlelight vigils and tourists who came to see the aftermath. The poster boards, photos and messages remained in place for several months even though we knew that the people in those photos and named in the messages were not going to return.

Life had to go on, so the photos and memorabilia came down. We didn't dare dispose of any of it, so it all went to storage along with the cards the staff received from the world over, including the three-foot long letter we received from the nurses who worked during the Oklahoma City bombing.

During the ER debriefings that followed, the common theme amongst the staff was frustration that we couldn't have done more—that we were ready to take a thousand more patients if we'd had to.

For a time thereafter, the majority of New Yorkers, myself included, feared taking the subways, and cringed at the sound of a plane flying overhead. I don't feel that way anymore. I refuse to live in fear.

A number of us left the ER. We went on to other forms of nursing, other hospitals, locations or jobs. There was a need to start over with a new practice, new faces, and a new perspective.

I appreciate my life and my family a lot more now. I live and plan for today. I say I love you every day to those I hold dear. I forgive the petty nonsense.

I will never forget the events of that day. I don't want to. It has strengthened my practice as a nurse and as a person. It gave me a unique perspective on how we, as nurses and rescuers, can come together in a time of crisis. When we are called upon to go beyond our scope, we can and we will. That's why we're in this job in the first place.

All of the disaster practice drills we go through as healthcare workers have value. We don't take it for granted. There is no sure-fire way to prepare us for what may happen in any given disaster—just ask the nurses in Oklahoma City, Saint Louis, Joplin and New York. What gets us through is what we already have inside us—that dedication which made us decide to be part of this profession in the first place.

STELLA

"After you get used to taking care of people in the ER, nothing really bothers you very much ever again."

I am seventy-five years old and I have been a nurse since 1943. I was raised during the Great Depression and watched my mother struggle to feed, shelter and clothe us kids. This was a good thing, because it gave me knowledge of what true suffering was like.

During World War II, the government offered women free education under the Cadet Nursing Program. We were dirt poor, so I jumped at the chance. I started out in a small town hospital in Minnesota, under the supervision of nuns. When I graduated from the nursing program, I remained at that hospital.

Private rooms back then cost thirteen dollars a day. Everything we used, we reused if possible and did our own autoclaving. At night I'd have thirty patients all mixed in together with just one 40-watt bulb over the nurse's desk. We didn't have penicillin yet, so I saw a lot of people die who, only one year later, could have been saved.

When I married, we moved to an Appalachian coal-mining town in West Virginia. That was where my real nursing education began. I took a job in the hospital, which was just an old hotel. Even though I lost fifteen pounds in the first few months just from worrying so much, it was a fantastic experience working in those hills. Never in my life had I seen anything like what went on there.

I was the only trained nurse in that so-called hospital. Nothing was ever sterilized, and there was barely anything to clean the basic instruments with. We did have a small operating room, but for those who were unfortunate enough to have surgery there, only a few survived. It was a daily occurrence for operations to be done on the wrong people. I remember a man who had a craniotomy after he'd come in with appendicitis, and the woman who had her gallbladder out when she'd come in for a hernia repair.

This was at a time when there was never any diagnosis written on the chart. Actually, there was rarely anything written in the chart other than the patient's name and maybe what medicines he was supposed to have.

In the back of the hotel was an old Victorian house that was an annex of sorts where the black folks went to be cared for. No white nurses were allowed to go back there, so self-trained black women were brought up from somewhere down south.

We had a black orderly named Harvest Moon who was one of the sweetest men alive. One stormy night the roof of the Annex caved in, so we sent Harvest over to see if he could help those poor souls. When he came back a few hours later, I asked him if anyone got hurt.

"Well yes," he answered. "But they was already dead."

Usually I worked alone, taking care of forty to fifty patients with ten more out in the hall. It was during this period of time that I had the worst experience of my whole career.

A woman came down from the back hills to deliver her baby. That by itself was pretty darned unusual to begin with, because those backwoods people almost never came down to us for anything. When it came time to deliver her baby, this thing came out of her that was, well, I don't know a better way to describe it other than to say it resembled a sweet potato. There were no limbs, and only a small bud-like thing for a head. No eyes or nose, no facial features except a tiny hole where the mouth should have been.

But it could cry, and cry it did, because it was hungry. I remember clearly the doctor pointing his finger at me and saying, "Don't feed it. Let it die."

So, I listened to that baby cry until it died. I can't recall anything about how the mother reacted. I just remember seeing that sweet potato lying there all wrapped up in a blanket and crying.

We really were primitive back then. Before the 1970s, the nurses were not expected, indeed, not allowed, to have anything to do with a man's private parts. Well, one of our frequent customers was a handsome young man who was always getting himself drunk and into trouble.

One night this man got into an automobile wreck and was brought in for observation. During the night he had to urinate, and couldn't navigate very well on account of being drunk and injured. I firmly believed there wasn't a patient I couldn't handle all by myself, so I helped him into the bathroom and held his penis while he urinated.

Well, you would have thought I'd run down the street stark naked the way the other nurses sneered at me. No one ever let me forget that, and it didn't help my cause one bit that every time he came in after that, he'd come through that door hollering for me. His calling for me had more to do with the fact that so many of the other nurses had such contempt for him, they treated him cruelly.

When the ICU and the ER were put into place, no one knew how to use the monitors or any of that other fancy equipment. Before 1970, the emergency room was just an extension of the operating room; there was no formal thing known as an emergency room.

Even though I could pretty much tell what was wrong with a patient just by looking at him, I learned how to run the monitors and the other fancy equipment, and in turn taught the doctors and the other nurses. It was nice, but I really didn't need all that fancy stuff.

Right up until about 1975, Dr. H, one of the old time physicians, used to come in and deliver babies barehanded, without so much as washing his hands first. We also had a young doctor who was an addict and used to go into the narcotic cabinet sometimes two or three times a night and take out however much Demerol he wanted. That was before the narcotic controls came in. Of course, he was dead at thirty-four, but that sort of thing used to happen quite a bit.

I remember so many little bits and pieces of things that happened, like the man who was in an automobile accident and had been burned to a crisp. Back then, in that part of the country there was no such thing as a morgue, so all the bodies came to us. In my mind's eye, I can still see the doctor putting a speculum between two of the deceased driver's ribs. The moment he started to open the speculum, the whole chest cracked into pieces, like a smashed up walnut shell. He took out the heart, which still had some non-congealed blood in it—for the blood alcohol test.

There was a lot of other nonsense going on too with women fretting over boyfriends or husbands who went off with other women. Once abandoned, those gals would take everything in the medicine chest in order to kill themselves, and we'd have to do a gastric lavage of charcoal and water.

Of course we dressed ourselves in expectation of the result, which was for the patient to throw up that black mud all over us. What a mess all that was. You'd think they would have just jumped in the river and be done with it.

My career came to an abrupt end when I was fifty-four. My youngest son, who was then twenty-six and newly married, was fatally burned in an industrial accident. When I looked at him in that burn unit, and knew there was nothing I could do for him, something broke inside me that never got put right again. I tried to go back to work, but I just couldn't see all those other sick people and not see my son lying in that bed.

Nursing did give me the knowledge of how to work through the grief eventually. Through the years, I'd seen plenty of other people lose their children. I drew upon the parents who'd seen their only son break his neck on the high school football field, and the woman who lost two sons to muscular dystrophy within eighteen months of each other, only to lose her third and last son to a car wreck a short time later.

I'd watched people be defeated by their trials and tribulations in life, and I wasn't about to do that. You learn from those people.

Nursing changed me. Years of watching the sick taught me to understand that life is not perfect and everyone has serious problems. Having to deal with all those folks' suffering causes a great gathering of your own strength and makes a better person of you. It certainly makes for a good nurse.

LUCILLE YIP
St. Vincent's Hospital, ER Nurse
New York City resident

"For me, the draw of ER nursing is the idea that we are jacks-of-all-trades. We see medical, surgical, trauma, obstetrics and gynecology, pediatric, psych and everything in-between. We see a constantly changing population of patients and never really know what's coming in next. You have to be on your toes every second—especially in New York City."

New York City
September 9, 2001
3 a.m.

Woke from a sound sleep. I don't know why, but I don't feel right. I'm too uneasy for sleep. Forty-four floors above lower Manhattan, I look out our living room window, and gaze at the spectacular New York skyline, full of lights and skyscrapers. The sight never fails to fill me with peace. I go back to bed at 5:30 a.m.

September 11, 2001
9:03 a.m.

I arrived home from a twelve-hour shift in the ER and fall into a deep sleep around 8 a.m. An hour later, the sound of an explosion wakes me. It isn't a garbage truck or a car crash—this is different. I've never heard anything like it in my life. Right away, I know something bad has happened.

I turn on the TV, and it takes a few seconds for the image of the World Trade Towers in flames to register in my mind. I don't believe what I'm seeing, so I run to my living room to see them with my own eyes. There they are—burning out of control in real time. From the TV I hear the newscasters say that planes have hit the towers, and I automatically think that terrorists have attacked us. There are several helicopters hovering over the buildings, including mine.

I call my sister, Anna, at the Federal Building. She answers and says only two words, "I'm leaving" and hangs up.

My husband calls to make sure I'm okay. I tell him I'm leaving for the ER and I probably won't be home tonight. He says, "Go. Go do what you have to do."

9:59 a.m.

I'm putting on my shoes, still watching out the window when I see the South Tower collapse like a house of cards. I sit frozen in stunned disbelief. The North Tower goes down 29 minutes later. Transfixed by the sight, I fall into a numb, shocky state of mind, and snap out of it only when the building super comes to the door to say the building must be evacuated because they don't know how many more planes are coming.

I go back to the window and stare out at my backyard that has turned into a war zone, then call my husband who is safe in Queens. All I say is, "The towers are gone."

Approximately 10:40 a.m.

I am running through Chinatown toward St. Vincent's Hospital, when I see hundreds of Wall Street people covered in white soot, walking toward me with that look on their faces—like the zombies in *The Night of the Living Dead*. Ambulances are speeding by coated in the same white soot, and I wonder what that stuff is. Cars parked along the streets all have their doors open and the radios blasting the news. Groups of New Yorkers are gathered around listening. On their faces I see what I feel. This can't be happening.

At Sixth Avenue, I realize it will take another forty minutes to get to St. Vinnie's if I have to continue on foot. I see a man with a sanitation logo on his car and I think, *He won't kill me because he works for Sanitation.*

I go over to explain to him that I'm a nurse trying to get to St. Vinnie's, and could he please give me a ride. There isn't one second of hesitation—he tells me to hop in.

St. Vincent's Emergency Room
10:50 a.m.

All around me is controlled chaos. It seems like St. Vincent's entire ER staff is present, along with nurses from other floors as well as nurses I recognize from other hospitals. Many of the nurses, like myself, left the ER just hours ago and have returned to help.

I am told the first wave of survivors, the majority of which were burn patients, cardiac arrests and crush injuries, have been treated and transferred upstairs.

What I'm seeing is the second wave of survivors and first-responder EMS workers. Most are suffering from smoke inhalation, eye injuries, lacerations from flying debris, and sprains and fractures sustained while running from the buildings. All of them are covered in that white soot. Like the people I saw in Chinatown, they all have that glazed look about them. There is no crying or screaming, just that disbelieving shocky stare and that weird quiet everywhere.

I am assigned to Unit Three, but there are so many nurses there already, I ask Suzanne Pugh, my manager, for permission to go out front to "The Cage," which is what we call our triage area. Jay Civello is the only nurse out there, and I figure he'll need help.

Across the street, the news media has lined up their cameras. CNN, BBC, and all the other news anchors are standing around hoping for a glimpse of survivors.

In triage I have to see every patient who enters the ER. I ask the ambulance people what the problem is with the patient, and when they tell me, I direct the patient to the appropriate area for care. Smoke inhalation and burns to the eyes I send to Unit Three. Crushed chest and skull fracture go to Unit Five. No names, no history, no vital signs. Nothing else—just the medical problem.

There is a team of ten or more registration people who stand in a line, each one armed with a clipboard and pen, waiting to follow them inside to record names and other information.

Suzanne comes outside, and Jay calls out, "Hey, Suzanne! We get time and a half for this, right?" It makes us all laugh for the first time all day. It's just what we need.

Approximately 3 p.m.
Where are the patients? We've not received any more survivors and the silence is deafening. All the nurses and doctors have been told we cannot leave the hospital until further notice, or until we know if the night staff will be able to get to us. The injured police coming in tell us that bridges, tunnels, buses and the subways are all closed down, so I don't know how the other staff people will get here to relieve us.

A part of me knows there won't be any more survivors, but a part of me is hoping there might be someone. Maybe they'll hear someone under the rubble and pull them out.

4 to 6 p.m.
Family members have been coming in by the hundreds looking for their loved ones. They all have the sound of desperation. This is the hardest thing for me, harder than watching that young firefighter die, harder than seeing the burns, harder than witnessing the towers collapse.

I am the first one they see. They look into my eyes hoping I will say, "Yes, your husband is here. He's on The List." But I don't get a chance to say that, because they are never on The List.

The List is my bible. It's the name of every patient in every hospital in the area—Beth Israel, New York Downtown, Bellevue, and Cornell Burn Center. It is updated every thirty minutes. The bad part is that every patient in every hospital is accounted for. There are no

John or Jane Does. Not one. This must be the first time in history that there have been no John or Jane Does after a disaster.

A young Hispanic woman asks me if her husband has come to our ER. I tell her no, and that I'm sorry. She says that when the first plane hit, she was working in the North Tower. Her husband, who worked in the South Tower, called to see if she was okay. She told him she was just leaving the building, and has not heard from him since.

She looks pale, tired and drained, as if she has not taken sustenance in days. It is exactly how I feel.

6:30 p.m.

A middle-aged woman comes in to say someone has posted her missing husband's name on the internet, along with the information that he is at St. Vincent's and that he's okay. I tell her that he isn't here. She insists he is, and shows me the computer printout. I show her The List.

She asks me where she should go. I tell her to go to the New School, where, I've been told, there are counselors who can talk to her. I don't tell her to go to the morgue, because I can't bring myself to say the words.

I want to break down and cry, but I can't, not now. I realize that I've not eaten or used the bathroom. I'm not hungry at all. Running on adrenaline, I guess.

A bright spot: my mother calls to say my sister is safe.

Approximately 6:30 – 8 p.m.

I think I would feel better if I could be in patient care doing something—starting an IV, bandaging—anything that would fix the problem. Being in triage, I can't do anything to fix the problem.

In nursing we are taught there is the short-term and long-term diagnosis. In triage there is no long-term diagnosis, except to tell someone their family member is in critical condition or a patient at the hospital.

I have such a sense of helplessness. For as crazy as working in ER is, I've always felt in control of my patients. Things simply are a certain way—if someone comes in with congestive heart failure, I'm going to give a little Lasix and they'll urinate and they'll feel better. If someone has a laceration, we'll clean it and suture it and it heals and it's fine. It's a universal recipe that works the majority of the time, but today, there is no recipe card for me to follow.

For the girl looking for her brother, there is nothing I can do but hug her and tell her how sorry I am. The nursing textbooks didn't teach us how to deal with such horrific tragedies.

8:45 p.m.

The night shift has arrived—all of them. I'm amazed that they have been allowed through.

I walk outside and find the streets empty. Barricades block off every intersection. All the stores and restaurants are closed. People are wearing facemasks. Everywhere there is smoke and more of that eerie silence.

I ask the driver of a police van filled with officers to give me a ride. He gladly complies and drops me off at Varick and Canal Streets, leaving me with a twenty-minute walk to my building. As I walk through the streets of lower Manhattan, I feel like my spirit has been sucked out of me and ripped into pieces. I am consumed by the silence, smoke, and the emptiness. Is this *my* New York?

A woman passes me wearing a facemask. We exchange stares, sharing the common grief, shock and disbelief. It is at that moment that I realize my life and the world as I know it have been changed forever.

A cop stops me and asks where I'm going. I tell him I need to get home. He asks to see some ID and when I show him my hospital ID, he says, "Get some rest. We're all in this together."

9:15 p.m.

My apartment smells like smoke. After my shower, the nextdoor neighbor brings food and encourages me to eat. To be polite, I nibble a little, but it turns to sawdust in my throat. I stay glued to the TV, unable to keep from watching the horrific pictures on the screen. I wish my husband were home.

September 12, 2001
2 a.m.

Can't sleep. The sound of the explosion still echoes in my head. It won't go away.

5 a.m.

I wake up in a cold sweat. The phone lines are down and I still can't reach my husband in Queens.

7 a.m.

I hitch a ride from two cops. They look angry and upset. At first I think they're angry with me for hitching a ride, and then I overhear one of them on his cell phone. He must be talking to his wife because he says, "Honey, I just came from Ground Zero. You can't believe what they did to us."

At work, most of the staff is just standing around waiting. I'm assigned to triage again. Maybe I'm lucky to be in triage. It's better than standing around. At least I get to help the families.

3 p.m.

Lots of firefighters come in with breathing problems secondary to smoke inhalation. We're seeing rescuers with burns to their eyes, open skull fractures, and fractures of the femur.

Throughout the day, the families continue to come in looking for family and friends. I continue to give the standard answer, "I'm sorry, she's not here. I'm sorry, he's not here. I'm sorry. I'm sorry." I can't remember how many times I've had to say that. It is breaking my spirit.

They all have that look that begs, "Please help me," and I'm not able to help except to touch a hand or give a hug. It feels like such an empty offering, but it's all that I can give.

Everywhere I look are tables of donated food and beverages. We even have massage therapists giving the staff free massages. Things are pretty quiet otherwise.

I talk with a police officer who was at Ground Zero. He tells me that most of the bodies are decapitated and the medical examiners are unable to determine the sex or race of the bodies.

I ask how he is holding up, and he says, "I haven't seen my kids. I'm exhausted. I don't know how I'm going to get over this."

8 p.m.

I hitch a ride home with a volunteer and we are detoured to the West Side Highway. Lining the road are crowds cheering for rescue workers, NYPD and us. They hold up signs that read: YOU ARE OUR HEROES!

But I don't feel like a hero. What have I done that anyone else wouldn't have done? Hero? Not at all.

8:30 p.m.

My husband is home and we hug each other for a long time. I go into the bathroom and sit on the side of the tub and cry hysterically. I start screaming, "God, what the hell were you thinking? I don't understand why you allowed this evil."

My husband comes in and sits with me, tears in his eyes. He doesn't try to tell me it will be okay. He doesn't try to tell me anything like that, and for this I am grateful.

9:30 p.m.

I look out my window and there are no lights. No skyline. There's just a cloud of smoke that covers what once was the World Trade Center. The depth of sadness is inexplicable.

September 13, 2001
6 a.m.

I sleep three hours. I have no desire for sleep or food. Instead, I watch TV and listen to the stories about the last calls made by passengers on the planes. I am overcome with emotion, and call my head nurse to see if I can come in early.

8 a.m. – 8 p.m.
I arrive in the ER after receiving a ride from the cops. I'm assigned to Unit Five, the critical care area of the ER. We are prepared for any survivors. The silence is deafening and maddening.

9 p.m.
I have to do something, so I ask a policeman to take me to Ground Zero. He parks the car somewhere near there. It's smoky, muddy, and I'm wearing my clogs. Within minutes, my feet are covered with that white mud. We don't walk very far when the cop says, "Here we are."

I look around and don't recognize anything. I ask, "Where are we?"

He looks at me funny and says, "Across the street from the World Trade Center." Then he asks if I'm going to be okay. I tell him of course I will, but as soon as he leaves, I know I'm not at all okay.

I stand there for a long time staring at what used to be the entryway. I stare at the mountain of rubble. I know it's crazy, but I'd been hoping that the buildings were still going to be there, but they aren't.

I walk around feeling like nothing is real. All the desks, chairs, buildings, and cars are crushed and covered with white dust. All the stores where I shop are gone. I keep walking, trying to force it to seem real. The only thing that is real is that my feet are full of mud.

One surreal scene after another presents itself as I walk around. I watch as the National Guard march in perfect lines—left, right, left, right—all by themselves, while behind them, rescue workers search for body parts.

I finally find the MASH unit and sign up to volunteer the next day. I walk back to Ground Zero. Transfixed by the sights of crushed cars, and the swarms of rescue workers and the faint smell of beginning putrefaction, I say good-bye to innocence and what life used to be.

A volunteer, a man named John, stops to ask if I'm okay and gives me a hug. That's when I break down and cry. He reads something in my face because he very gently leads me to St. Paul's chapel, located not too far from the World Trade Center.

I'm surprised the chapel isn't damaged. All the windows are in perfect condition. There are many volunteers there seeking refuge and comfort.

I walk into the dark chapel and sit in the pew. I begin to sob for the hundreds of times I have said, "I'm sorry, he's not on The List." I weep for the firefighter who was crushed. I weep for the dead.

When I leave, John takes the engraved wooden cross from around his neck, presses it into my hand, and says, "God bless you, my dear." He is such a light in this whole dark tragedy, and I am grateful for him.

Walking home, people stop to ask if I'm okay and to say thank you. I don't understand. Thank you? For what?

September 14, 2001
Approximately 3 p.m.

I'm assigned to Unit Five again. Rumors abound. We hear that six firefighters have been found alive in the rubble. We get excited and clear everyone out of Unit Five. We get the equipment ready, but no firefighters come.

Then we hear there is a pregnant woman found under the rubble and she is coming to us—but there isn't any pregnant woman. It's like a roller coaster ride.

Enough already. I convince myself that there are no survivors. No one down there is alive anymore.

February 18, 2002

I'd like to think I've become more compassionate and understanding of people since that day. It has made me rethink my purpose on this earth. I truly believe my purpose is to do the best I can to make a positive difference in other people's lives.

I've seen the dark side of people and I've seen the wonderfulness of people wanting to help each other. I've fallen in love with New Yorkers again—they all pulled together. It didn't matter what race or class anyone was. We were all under attack and we stuck together.

I haven't been back to Ground Zero. I didn't start reading the New York papers until just two weeks ago. I have no desire to watch any of the specials on TV. The pain is still very raw and I need to heal. But, like the other nurses, I feel I need to put up a good front. None of us have spoken about it to each other yet.

Letters and cards of gratitude from all over the country still cover the walls of the ER and it helps ease our pain. The ER is starting to feel normal again. No more cameras, no more reporters, and our frequent flyers have all returned.

Our weekly drug-addicted patients have all come back to St. Vinnie's to roost. It's actually "normal" now that I see Mr. G arriving to the ER under the influence, and verbally abusing us by chanting, "Shut the fuck up, shut the fuck up, shut the fuck up." He has such a rhythm going, we all have a good laugh and then we stop hearing him after a while. When he asks me to marry him, I smile and realize that despite the horrific tragedy, people have moved on with their every day lives.

Yeah, I think it's going to get better now. Life is headed back to normal.

December, 2014

Every year I take the time to honor and remember those who died during 9/11. Thirteen years have passed and I can still remember the sounds and smells of that day as if it were yesterday.

To this day, I am unable to watch any anniversary media footage on 9/11. I have not visited Ground Zero, nor do I have a desire to do so in the future. The healing process has been slow and perhaps one day I'll be able to see the Memorial.

I've learned so much from my experiences on 9/11. I treasure the time when I was able to make a difference in people's lives. I've learned that God can take the broken pieces in my life and make them into masterpieces.

I am blessed to live on Maui with my eleven-year-old son. He often asks about my personal experience as the 9/11 anniversary approaches, and I tell him that I would not have wanted to be anywhere else but New York during that time. I want him to understand how fortunate we are to live in a country that offers such great opportunities despite the tragedies in history.

I am glad to be able to tell my story about what happened that day. Nurses are often in the background working tirelessly, but the satisfaction of being able to help others, far outweighs the lack of recognition.

ROBIN

"There are people who are born ER nurses, but I'm definitely not one of them. I find ER medicine boring. Yeah, yeah, I know—it's chaotic and you have no control over what's going to come in, which is supposed to be exciting, but after a while, you see a lot of the same stuff over and over. ICU nursing is much more autonomous in terms of problem solving. In the ICU you're on your own. In ER I never really felt I was using my judgment or my skills, so a month ago, I gave notice. I'll be starting in the ICU next week.

"Since today was my last shift in ER, I'm going to give you a running account of everything that happened from the time I walked in until I left. Keep in mind that this shift was a carbon copy of the day before and the day before that—just different players.

"I hope when I'm finished, you'll understand why I'm leaving the ER far behind me."

At 8 a.m. I'm out of the nurses' locker room dressed in scrubs that I know when I take them off, will be covered with other people's bodily fluids. This is mainly due to the fact that it is the nurses who are responsible for running the three trauma bays—medical, acute and pediatric.

My first duty of the day is to check and restock the twenty-four treatment rooms. I then call the three triage desks out front—acute, non-acute and ambulance—to see if there's anything cooking. I'm told there are eighteen patients in non-acute waiting to be seen, and more are coming in the door. I know what these patients will look, sound, and smell like. Most will be druggies looking for three hots and a cot, some will be legitimate sprains and cuts and small traumas.

I check the staffing—eight nurses, two attendings, two residents, three rotating residents from other hospitals, and what seems like way too many interns and medical students.

As I am walking to the treatment room to help with a dislocated shoulder, I hear someone pounding on the door that goes out to the ambulance bay. I ignore it, passing it off as kids fooling around, but then I hear shouts and a man screaming, "Oh Jesus, help me!"

I open the side door and a man falls forward onto his face, a knife sticking out of his back. It's like a scene out of a movie. For a nanosecond, I study the position of the knife and try to figure out what organs have most likely been affected. I do a quick, overall assessment, and see that he's bleeding profusely from multiple stab wounds. I'm amazed he's still breathing. I recognize the man. He is one of our frequent flyers and HIV positive to boot.

I yell for help and ten seconds later, four of us pick him up and get him onto a gurney. The trauma surgeon, one of the old school military types, is barking orders as we head down the hall to the acute trauma bay. As we approach the trauma bay door, the surgeon sticks his ungloved hand inside the patient's chest to stop the bleeding and insists we head straight for the OR. I inform him that the guy is HIV positive, but he gives no indication of having heard me nor does he stop and glove up.

When I return to the ER, I see one of our nurses rubbing a fresh welt on her bare leg and I know Roger is here. Roger is one of our regular drunks. He comes in about four times a week carrying a cane with which he assaults the nurses and security guards. He has injured hospital personnel so severely as to put a few in the hospital.

In order to get him from the stretcher to the gurney, we need two EMS guys, Jon, who is our only male RN on staff, and three security men to get him over. Today Roger scores by kicking Jon full-force in the groin.

Jon drops cold to the floor. Secretly, I'm disappointed that it isn't one of the EMS guys instead, since it's a felony to assault an EMS worker, but only a misdemeanor to assault a doctor or a nurse. We would love to nail this sucker to the walls of the county jail and leave him there to dry.

I check to make sure Jon is still breathing then wheel him to the back nurses' lounge where I give him an ice pack to hold between his legs until a doc can see him and write an order for him to go home.

Ambulance triage rings to tell us that we're getting a code three shooting victim in full arrest. I run to the trauma bay just as the stretcher wheels in. The patient is a twenty-year-old female who walked out of a convenience store in the projects at the wrong time. Some gangbangers were doing a little target practice and got her in the head and chest.

The paramedics tell us she had moved from the neighborhood three years ago to get away from the violence, but came back to visit her mother. She has no chance of survival, but because of her age and the fact a bystander said she was pregnant, the paramedics began CPR and brought her to us.

I see the ragged bloody hole in the left temporal area, and when I move around to the other side of the stretcher to pull her onto the gurney, I stop cold. The woman's upper right chest and shoulder are completely blown away. Bits of rib and tissue are scattered all over her as the blood flows down over the mound of her pregnant belly like a river.

The OB team brings in the ultrasound, and sure enough, there is the five-month-old fetus struggling desperately to stay alive. It makes me sick to watch, so I turn away. One of the other nurses breaks the silence that has fallen over the room and says, "Well, we sure as hell can't go home and talk to our family about *this* one."

An intern says that we should have the chaplain come down to say a few words, but nobody pays any attention because another ambulance has arrived and is delivering a patient to the trauma bay next door.

I walk into the room and see an elderly white woman in her seventies. Despite the fact that the top of her skull is missing, she is awake and talking pleasantly, as if she were having tea instead of major trauma. There is a sliver of glass sticking to the surface of her partially exposed brain, and I wonder whether or not I should pick it off as one might pick off a piece of lint from someone's jacket.

I introduce myself and while I am preparing sterile towels soaked in saline to cover the bared gray matter, I ask her name, address, the date, and the name of the president, all of which she answers correctly.

I press the doctor call button three times, a signal that means STAT—Latin for statum, or, immediately. Her blood pressure is mostly okay at one hundred over forty. I'm preparing to insert a large-bore intravenous catheter into the woman's vein when the woman points to the elderly well-dressed gentleman sitting in the corner.

"That's my husband, George," she says. "We've been married fifty-two years."

George hobbles slowly to the gurney, and lays a hand tenderly on his wife's stick-thin leg. Behind Coke bottle lenses, his rheumy blue eyes look huge and frightened.

"We were driving to choir practice at St. Hillary's over on Second and Mission," he begins, and I get the feeling he's trying to convince himself he's not dreaming. "I was at the bottom of the hill when along comes a fella in one of those cement trucks and sideswipes Judy's side of the car. I never saw him coming."

A string of spit flies from his mouth. He pulls a snow-white linen handkerchief from his breast pocket and wipes the spittle off his chin. He seems to lose his train of thought for a moment, then resumes. "I checked to see if she was okay. There was blood everywhere, but I couldn't tell where it had come from. I tried wiping some of it off, and I'll be damned if right there on the seat were these—" He moves his hands side to side, as if sifting for the right word, "—two big pieces of Judy's noggin with the hair still attached!

"I picked them up and set them right back on top of her head."

"Like a beanie cap," his wife says.

"More like a jigsaw puzzle," George says.

They both cover their mouths and giggle like children. He kisses her cheek as tears well in his eyes.

"She's my girl," he says, "I'm just happy she's alive. I don't know what I'd to do without her."

My patient smiles up at him adoringly then freezes for a split second before her eyes roll back in what is left of her head. She begins to seize as I hustle him out of the room, yelling for a code blue.

At once, her vital signs all head south. A piece of brain matter falls onto the top of my shoe and I wonder what part of her body or thoughts it controlled. Perhaps, I think, it's the part that made her sing on key.

Later, when I can face it, I go to the meditation room, which is where we put the survivors, to speak with the husband.

When I tell him we could not save her, he repeats, "I can't believe she's gone." about ten times before the hospital chaplain takes over.

I wonder how the new widower will get home, and what he'll do once he gets there. Will he chose her clothes for the mortician, or will he go to bed? How will he sleep his first night in fifty-two years without her?

I don't think about this too long, because the trauma triage desk calls to say we have four stabbing victims in the waiting room.

I hustle toward the lobby and see four teenage girls in wheelchairs. They have been involved in all-girl gang warfare with a rival gang. Each is moaning and holding some part of her body—breast, neck, arm and abdomen.

I do a cursory check of each girl's wound and take back the one stabbed in the arm since her brachial artery has been nicked, and she's going into shock from the loss of blood. Knowing that she's going to need blood, I order a stat type and crossmatch, and situate her on a gurney before calling in the attending.

I'm surprised to see it's after noon. By the time I actually make it to the bathroom, my bladder is floating up around my teeth and tears are welling in my eyes. The nurses' toilet is occupied, so I hurry to the lobby restroom. I'm halfway across the lobby when I see a flash of blue out of the corner of my eye a nanosecond before the retort of the gunshot reaches my ears.

A woman screams and I consider whether or not I should just keep heading to the restroom, or drop to the floor. At the thought of stopping, my bladder lets go of a few drops as a warning.

Another gunshot rings out, and I hit the terrazzo floor, sliding the rest of the way to the ladies' on my belly. I quickly relieve myself and open the restroom door a half-inch, listening for more gunfire. The only thing I hear is a woman's hysterical screams bouncing off the lobby walls.

Keeping low, I hunch over like Groucho Marx and make a beeline to the trauma bay where a man in his early twenties is undergoing some vigorous CPR. On one side of his head is a round purple hole and on the other, a crater the size of my fist. The monitor indicates he's in asystole—a flatliner. His pupils are blown, and I just can't get excited about flogging a corpse.

I pilfer a couple of Valiums from the nurses' private stockpile of meds, and go in search of the hysterical woman. She is easy to find—all I have to do is follow the trail of policemen. After checking to make sure she isn't the shooter, I tell the cops I need to get her calmed down. At the sight of my uniform and nametag, she grabs me, begging for news of the shooter's condition.

"He's not doing great," I say, leaving out the part that he's dead. "They're doing everything they can."

The girl, who looks to be about sixteen, but is in fact twenty-two, tells me the patient is her boyfriend. She informs me that he's been depressed ever since he lost his job two months ago. This morning he woke up and told her he was going to kill himself.

Not knowing what else to do, she'd driven him to the hospital. The two of them then sat in the ER parking lot for three hours while she begged him to sign himself in and get help.

When he finally agreed, she'd come into the lobby for a wheelchair. She was only a few yards from the car when he got out, shouted that he loved her, and pulled a gun from his boot. The first shot missed his head altogether. The second did not.

I want to empathize with her, but I can't. I want to tell her to move on and next time to make a better choice of men, but that's not okay either. Instead, I give her a Valium and leave her to the police.

I report off to the oncoming charge nurse and head to the locker room to change. As I peel off my scrub top, I don't bother trying to remember which patient's blood made each reddish brown or magenta stain. I stopped doing that years ago.

As I shower, I try to imagine that every horrific tragedy I have witnessed over the last five years, is being washed out of my memory and disappearing down the drain. All those faces full of suffering, all the battered or dead children, all the evidence of hate, prejudice and cruelty—washed away and gone.

OLGA

"Nurses get a little left of center when they work ER for an extended period of time. I think it's because, when things get right down to the nitty-gritty, we get a really unique and weird view of humanity."

I guess I felt bad for the guy, which is why I started paying more attention to him. He was obviously uncomfortable the way he kept squirming around, flushed and sweating, and wearing that weird expression.

Ever since he signed in, he'd been calling someone every few minutes, but as far as I could tell, no one had returned his call.

Romantic that I am, I imagined the whole sad story: A tearful argument, then his lover slamming out the door, deserting him in his hour of need, gone off with another Village boy.

Our ER is located right in the middle of a large gayborhood, so we get a lot of gay men. We've seen it all and heard it all. Nothing is shocking or new to the nurses who work here. I've personally seen all manner of things pulled from the anal sphincters of our gay patients: tennis balls (because they're collapsible), full Heineken bottles (because they fizz in just the "right" way), Barbie doll heads (because they feel good coming out). I've always wanted to ask, "Why not *Ken?*"

Having noted that the poor guy was getting glassy-eyed while he squirmed, I brought him back to the treatment area. I took his pressure, which was high, and his pulse, which was racing. I didn't really want to, but it's part of my job to find out what the foreign body was that was up there. I finally asked, praying that it wasn't a mammal, a reptile, or some kind of sharp object that could perforate his bowel.

He answered in a low, whispery voice, so I could barely hear him. However, I was pretty sure he'd said "peeper."

Thinking of fuzzy yellow chicks, I opened my mouth to ask how many of the little fowls he'd managed to insert, when a distant buzzing reached my ears. The sound and rhythm was familiar.

I held up a hand. "Shhh," I said, listening really hard. "What's that sound?"

My patient didn't answer because he was in what looked to be the throes of an orgasm. Only then did it dawn on me. Beeper. He'd put his beeper on vibrate mode, inserted it and was paging himself into oblivion.

As sick as it was, I realized right then and there that it is exactly this sort of thing that keeps me going to work every day.

ANGEL LOPEZ
Ground Zero
Hospice nurse, Tucson, Arizona

"*I went into nursing because I was raising a family and I needed the money. I started out as an OR nurse, but when one of my good friends was dying of AIDS, I had my first exposure to hospice nursing. I am a spiritual person, and death is a spiritual experience no matter what your belief system. I've been hooked on hospice nursing ever since.*

"*I have lupus and a whole list of autoimmune disorders. Early in 2001, my doctor told me that I didn't have much time left to live because my immune system was shutting down. One of the things I wanted to do before I died was to make a road trip around the United States.*

"*I did a lot of meditating and self-healing, and at the end of June, I felt the spirits telling me to hit the road and go to Prince Edward Island, Canada. I sold everything I had and left my family and home on July 9, 2001. I drove across the United States and Canada on a ten thousand mile trip that was to become the most spiritual journey of my life.*

"*Late on September 9, I drove into Prince Edward Island. On September 10, I spent an absolutely glorious day basking nude in the Atlantic Ocean, convinced I'd died and gone to heaven. On*

September 11, the lady from the hostel where I was staying woke me to say that something bad had happened to America. As soon as I heard the news, I knew why I'd been given the message to hurry."

September 14, 2001
Prince Edward Island, Canada

I couldn't get out of Canada for three days because all the borders were sealed. As soon as they opened, I drove a thousand miles in twenty-four hours. I'd never been to New York before—hell, I'd never even been east of the Mississippi. I didn't have any money left and I didn't have a place to go, so I just followed what the Spirits wanted me to do.

At 9:30 a.m., I drove into Manhattan and went right to Bellevue hospital. I actually found a parking space in front of the Wall of Prayer—which, I am told, was a miracle in and of itself. I walked into the hospital and told a nurse that I was a hospice nurse and I was there to help.

I was directed to the emergency room where one of the physicians provided me the address of the Javits Center. I got back in the car and drove there, walked through all the security people without anyone stopping me, and signed in. As I looked around, I realized that nobody really knew what the hell they were doing. It was a mess. There was no organization, and everybody wanted to be in charge.

That was when I saw Ann Carroll for the first time. She and another nurse were in a buzz about straightening up the first aid station and labeling boxes. There are people who really need to do that type A stuff. Personally, I'd rather talk to the cute guys. At the time, I didn't say anything to Ann, mainly because the woman never sat down.

By nightfall there were only four nurses left—me, Ann, a nurse from Ohio, and one from Manhattan. All of us were independent nurses who wanted to give our help where it was needed the most but none of us had Ground Zero access. Also, the Red Cross was going through all this insane brouhaha about who was in charge.

The four of us decided we didn't want to play that game, so we went to the FEMA office and said that we were there to relieve the nurses down at Ground Zero. They bought our story without question, and within ten minutes, gave us FEMA and EMS badges and a police escort down to Ground Zero. They dropped us off and there we were.

We hadn't been down at Ground Zero very long when the nurse from Manhattan had to leave because she wasn't feeling well. The Ohio nurse wasn't physically fit and couldn't move as quickly as she needed to, so she dropped out. That left Ann and me to do walking triage.

We used Red Cross supplies and manned their stations when we were there, but mostly we were on our own. It wasn't until we left three weeks later that the Ground Zero officials began cracking down on doing background checks on exactly who everybody was. I hate to burst anybody's bubble, but security was a total illusion. Our intentions were loving, so for us, it all worked out for the best.

Ann and I called ourselves the walking triage unit. We carried medical kits and water and mostly tended to the workers' eyes, feet, respiratory problems and hydration. Each day Ann would tell me what our mission was going to be, and I went along. Our missions usually met the given need—one day it would be water, the next it would be insoles, the next, mask filters. Whatever was needed, we provided.

On our second night at Ground Zero, we entered the rubble of the World Trade Center. As we were walking around those unstable piles of what was left of the buildings, I realized the danger of being there and said to Ann, "You know that we may not get out of here alive, right?"

She said she knew, so then I asked, "What are we going to do?"

She answered, "We're going to do our jobs."

And that's what we did for three weeks straight.

The whole time we walked around on top of the rubble that was Ground Zero, we had the feeling that we were treading on souls. We didn't dare allow ourselves to feel while we were there. There was a sense that if we allowed ourselves to feel, we wouldn't be able to do our jobs. Only when I was away from Ground Zero did I allow myself to grieve. The people who were down there are still afraid to talk about their emotions because they're afraid to feel it. There are people who will never feel any of it.

I saw Ann's strength, and decided I'd do whatever I could until I couldn't do it anymore. The whole situation was bigger than me, and the only way I could get through it was to honor the Spirit.

As it turned out, I didn't need to be the nurse—Ann was the nurse from day one, and I was the loving energy that everyone needed. On the back and front of whatever shirt and hat I was wearing, I wore a sign that read, *I GIVE HUGS*.

The result of wearing that message was that I tapped into some incredible emotions. When we walked down the street, there wasn't a person who didn't want to give me a hug. Grown men and policemen would come to me for hugs. Guys driving dump trucks stopped traffic and jumped out of their trucks for a hug.

One day a priest came walking out of the temporary morgue looking pretty worn down. He saw my hat and asked for a hug. As I hugged him he said, "You cannot even imagine how many body parts I have blessed today."

I said, "There's nothing I can do about that, but I'll hold you for as long as you need me to."

One night at the Red Cross station I noticed something going on with a young crane operator who had been surrounded by mental health workers for a couple of hours. I was told that the mental health people wanted to put him in a psych unit for drug rehab because he'd taken a snort of cocaine.

Eventually someone came over and asked if I was the Hug Lady. I said I was, so they brought me over to this young guy. I didn't say anything except to turn and show him my shirt. Without hesitation, he took me in his arms, laid his head on my shoulder and started to talk.

"I took my scoop out of the rubble today," he said, "and there was a half a woman hanging from it. I'm just a crane operator, for God's sake! I can't do this!"

As soon as I heard that, I told the mental health workers to back off. To have seen the awful things he saw, I didn't blame him for snorting that coke. One of the mental health workers came up to me later and said, "You know, you did more for that kid in fifteen minutes than the rest of us did in the last two hours."

My intent while I was down at Ground Zero was to be a vessel of love and blessing. The energy that came to me from all the people I touched every day, didn't stay in me, it went *through* me in the sense of channeling their spirits. I took it in, and let it out to the universe. The energy was constant. I didn't take one step down at Ground Zero without praying regardless of whether I was trudging through the muck, irrigating eyes, tending to blisters, or hugging someone.

For the first two nights, Ann and I couldn't sleep. We were sleeping in the basement of the elementary school and when we finally lay down to try to get some sleep, everything hurt—every muscle and bone. We were exhausted. I remember helping Ann, who absolutely could not move without pain, and thinking, *What is wrong with this picture? Here's a healthy woman, and I'm taking care of* her? I realized then that the only way I could do what I was doing was because Spirit was in me.

About five or six days into our work at Ground Zero, the Red Cross could see that we were working ourselves to death and insisted we go to a spa down the street that was offering free services to rescue workers. It was the first time we were able to take hot showers. Ann just lay down on the couch and crashed. I went into the sauna and sobbed uncontrollably for about two hours. I couldn't stop. I cried for all those souls who died in fear, panic and chaos.

They had shifts of some fifty firefighters who would rotate in and out of Ground Zero every three hours, so there was always a group of men waiting outside the morgue to go in for their shift. I would go there and just sit with them.

One night, one of the younger firefighters told me that he didn't feel he could keep going into the rubble. I could see his pain so I asked him what his pain was all about.

"It's the kids," he said. "There were kids in the buildings and kids on the planes and those bastards didn't care about them. I don't understand how anybody could do that. When you got little kids at home, you can't understand it."

Ann and I used to visit the construction trailers down at the site to see if anyone needed anything. In one of the trailers was a photograph of a little girl tacked on the wall, so I asked the worker if it was his little girl.

"No," he replied. "That was found intact in the rubble. There's a lost parent somewhere in there. When we get tired and feel like we can't do this anymore, we come in here and look at this picture and that's what keeps us going."

Most of the people who worked at Ground Zero have been traumatized for life. During my time there, I saw that many of them were deep into the post-traumatic stress disorder thing and having all sorts of medical issues.

Toward the end, I got frustrated with Ann because she wouldn't stop. I told her I couldn't do it anymore, but she still wouldn't stop and I would not leave her—that would have been like cutting off my right arm. For the whole time we were down there, we were never apart for more than a few minutes.

I finally said, "Ann, we can't save the world. We have to stop now."

On our last day there was a memorial service on Hudson Bay for the firemen who died. I sat with my back to people so they could see my shirt. I ended up hugging family members all day long—wailing mothers who had lost their sons, pregnant women who'd lost their husbands, four tow-headed boys who'd lost their father.

In the past, I have been known to be a very angry and self-destructive person. I've been known to be engulfed by my own rage. What I realized at Ground Zero was that *that* kind of anger was exactly what produced Ground Zero. I understood that on a deep spiritual level, which is why I would not feed into the angry vengeance, the "nuke 'em, kill 'em" mentality of most of the workers. That was hard because I was in the minority.

I voiced my thoughts about non-violent forgiveness just once and was shunned immediately, so I knew I couldn't speak about it, but I could live it. I understood their pain, but I honored my own truth in being a loving presence in that anger.

I tell people that working at Ground Zero was one of the most traumatizing, one of the most devastating, and one of the most loving experiences of my life. For me it was a healing experience—an experience of absolute surrender and being in the moment. It was all about love, and love's divine power.

I am forever changed. Nothing bothers me anymore. I've not had one medical problem since, and I'm off all medications. My lab work is the best it's been in three years.

I don't feel like a hero. We all have jobs to do on this planet and this was just part of my job. I struggle with telling my story because there are no words to articulate the emotions. Ground Zero stories are a part of me. I don't need to write them down.

DARCY

"I've been in nursing for three years. I learned early on that one of the main requirements for being an ER nurse is that you must be extremely instinctual.

"Before I became a nurse, I wrote title insurance and worked for attorneys. When my youngest son was born with Hyaline Membrane Disease, I was so impressed with the nurses that I made the decision to quit my job and go to nursing school.

"At first I worked in labor and delivery, but after awhile I was bored to tears. I have a super-short attention span, so I have to have something going on all the time. An EMT friend of mine kept telling me that ER was the only way to go. One night he was killed in the ambulance going on a call, so I felt I owed it to him to find out if ER was for me.

"Then again, my dad was a paramedic for twenty-eight years. When he'd come home from work, he'd tell us stories that would have us glued to our chairs, so in a way, I guess his love of chaos rubbed off on me.

"It's the pace of the ER that I love. That, and being able to take people from death's door and bring them back to the land of the living. And if the patient dies despite what we do, I like being able to put the survivors back together enough to get on with life.

"All of that has its own reward, so here I am."

"Hi. I've got my handy little micro-recorder here, and I've decided that instead of doing a taped interview about my past ER experiences, I'd tape parts of my shift in real time, as I go through it.

"Right now it's about eight p.m., and I've just finished getting report on the patients who are in the waiting room and the ones who are already in the treatment rooms.

"We don't have anybody serious—two lacerations, a sprained ankle that needs splinting, a repeater scumbag in the drunk tank sleeping it off, and an eight-month-old who had a febrile seizure. The parents are more in need of help than the baby. This is their first kid, and you know how they can be—hysterics with a capital H.

"We've also got an old lady from Mt. View nursing home with a urinary tract infection, and a man visiting from China who has bleeding hemorrhoids. The woman in—"

(*In the background the EMS radio buzzes. A paramedic identifies himself as Callahan and says they are at the ER's backdoor with a seventeen-year-old male who was found unresponsive outside an apartment complex. The teen's parents have been notified and are on their way.*)

"Okay, folks, here we go." (*Sounds of running, doors opening, and general confusion.*)

"Oh okay. This kid looks okay. He's sitting up and talking.

"Hey Callahan, I thought you said the kid was unresponsive. This guy looks better than I do.

"Hey there, can you tell me your name?"

"Ray."

"Okay Ray, can you tell me why you're here?"

"I don't know. I got fucked up on some drugs I guess. I don't remember exactly."

"What kind of drugs?"

"Some rock. I smoked a little rock."

"You mean crack?"

"Yeah."

"Anything else?"

"I think I had a beer earlier."

"One beer and some crack? Is that all?"

"Yeah. Are my parents here?"

"Your mom and dad are on their way."

"Oh man, I hurt so bad."

"Where do you hurt?"

"I don't know. My belly, my back, my head. Everywhere. I've got a bad headache. I feel pretty sick. I think I'm gonna—"

"Here! Throw up in here. That's it. It's going to be okay. Why do you hurt? Did you fall or get into a fight or something?"

"Yeah."

"Yeah what?"

"I got into a fight with three dudes. They had baseball bats. They surprised me. I didn't know they were going to do anything—they just snuck up and started beating on me. I think I passed out."

(*The patient's parents and brother come into the room. Ray starts to cry. Tape stopped.*)

"Hi again. Well, Ray is on his way to surgery. I got a bad feeling as I was taking him to x-ray for belly films. He definitely started looking crummy. The resident came in to put in an NG tube, so I left him alone with the kid and when I came back in, the kid wasn't breathing.

"I got the attending to intubate him so we could get him in for a CT scan of his head. Turns out his skull was crushed, so we rushed him down to the OR. I haven't quite mastered the concept that just because they're talking to me doesn't mean there isn't something major going on. I hope the kid makes it. He seems like a good kid. He kept apologizing to his parents.

"I see these kids come in with their injuries and horror stories and it makes me paranoid. I don't even let my seven-year-old ride in the front seat anymore. I've seen eight and nine-year-olds come in DOA after a simple fender bender because they'd been riding in the front seat and the airbags inflated and killed them.

"I don't like taking care of the infants. Kids over a year and a half are okay; younger than that, I can't handle. They're just so tiny, I hate seeing them suffer."

(*In the background, the clerk tells her there's a woman in labor in the lobby.*)

"Okay, I've got a live one out in the lobby." (*Sounds of running.*) "Did I mention that I also hate delivering babies on an emergency basis? I swear that half the babies born in this town are delivered in the back seats of cars right here in our parking lot. Usually by the time Mom gets to our back door, the baby is already partially delivered. Then, you have to get the woman's underpants off immediately before they strangle the child.

"Where the hell is—? Excuse me, are you the—?"

"I am the husband." (*The man has a thick accent.*)

"It says here that you and your wife have been in the United States for only three months?"

"Yes. We are from Africa."

"Okay, follow me. Let's get mom to our obstetrics room. Does your wife, ah, Fatamina? Does she speak any English?"

"No English. I speak for her."

"Does she have a doctor here? Has she had any prenatal care?"

"No, no doctor in United States. In Africa, yes."

"Please explain to her that I need to take her skirt and underpants off. How long has she been in labor?"

"Ten hours."

"Ten hours? No, no. Don't be afraid, Fatamina. It's okay, I'm just going to check and see how far you are— Don't hit me, please. Fatamina, you need to let me—

"Um, sir? Would you explain to your wife that I need to examine her?"

(The husband speaks in a foreign language. The woman responds in a voice that is strained.)

"Okay, that's good. Thank you. All right, now try to relax and let me take a look here and see how far the baby—

"Oh dear. Ah, I, um. Excuse me, sir, but can you tell me what happened here?"

(The woman speaks rapidly and begins to shriek.)

"My wife, she was circumcised when she was young."

"She's—? You mean she's—? Okay. Okay. Hold on, I need to get the doctor. Please tell her to pant like this."

(Darcy pants until the woman joins her. Then there is the sound of running.)

"Hey, Dr. P, I need you in the OB room stat! I've got a woman in there who's been in labor for ten hours. The kid is crowning, but the woman has been circumcised. The opening is small and scarred—too small for the baby's head to get through. We need to get the kid out of there soon, or we're going to lose him."

(*The sound of a door opening. The woman is grunting and panting.*)

"Hello, I'm Dr. P. Let's see what we've got here. Darcy, get that light over here. We've got to—Oh shit! Darcy, you're going to have to help me do this."

(*Darcy yells over the sound of the woman screaming.*)

"We need to cut that right there, Dr. P."

"I'll knick the baby if I do that."

"Trust me, you won't. Here, take the scissors and do it like this. That's it. Okay, here he comes! That's it, that's it. Push, Fatamina. Good! One more. Okay, doc, get ready to grab him!"

(*There's a lot of commotion and the sounds of the woman straining to push. Then, the wail of a newborn. The husband is speaking rapidly to his wife. Tape is turned off.*)

"Hi, it's me again. I'm on a bathroom break. The good news is that the baby is fine. The bad news is that one of the OR techs just came down to tell us that Ray, the seventeen-year-old kid, died on the table.

"You know sometimes when I go home, I tell my husband all these stories, and he's fascinated by it. He says, "Wow, isn't it cool when that shit happens?" And I answer, "No, not really.""

(*Sound of a door opening and someone telling Darcy she needs to come out because the department is swamped.*)

"Okay, here we go again." (*Tape is turned off.*)

"Me again. Sorry but in the chaos I forgot to turn the tape back on. I'll try to recap what came in.

"First there was a freaky accident. A mom and dad were arguing at the dinner table. Dad, who was drunk off his ass, threw a plate at mom. The plate missed mom, hit the wall and shattered. A shard of china hit the teenage daughter in the temporal artery, severing it. She's in surgery now.

"As soon as I cleared that circus out, a sixty-five-year-old woman came in who accidentally put her hand in the shredder. She heard something clacking around inside the machine, and reflexively stuck her hand in to fix it.

"Her fingers looked like sliced luncheon meat. The most amazing thing was that the woman didn't react much. Her vitals were fine, and she was calm. Most people would have been coming off the ceiling.

"After that, a teenaged couple came in completely freaked out because the condom got lost inside the girl's vagina and they couldn't find it. We—"

(The sound of a door opening.) "Hey Darcy, you got a crazy guy in room fourteen. Here's his chart."

"Oh wow. This is going to be a good one. Here I go." *(Sounds of ER chaos in the background. She begins laughing.)*

"Oh my god. I can see the patient through the window and he's probably six-feet-three and weighs about two hundred pounds. He's got a whole roll of toilet paper wrapped around his head like a helmet.

"Hi, I'm Darcy. What seems to be the problem, Mr. um, Magical? Is Magical your real name?"

"Yeah, I'm Mr. Magical. I think I'm suicidal. I tried to kill myself with a nail gun."

"How about if I just take off all this toilet paper and see what you've got under there.

"Okay well, it seems there's six nails sticking out of the top of your head. This is how you tried to kill yourself?"

"Yeah, I guess so. I've got a bad headache. Can you give me something?"

"Well, the doctor has to take a look at this before I can give you anything. We'll bring you to x-ray and then you might have to go to surgery to get those nails out of there. Stay here and I'll get the doctor. Don't touch your head."

(Sound of the door opening and closing. Darcy laughs.) "Jesus. This reminds me of the woman who came in about a month ago complaining that she had something in her leg. She said she was getting in the car, and she felt something poke her in the knee, but she didn't know what it was.

"The x-ray showed a sixteen-inch meat skewer going through her knee and down into the calf muscle. I didn't make any sense to me, either, but I've learned not to ask too many questions." *(Tape is turned off.)*

"Hi, it's me again. Well believe it or not, I'm standing in our trauma room looking at a man's leg on a gurney. No man—just his leg. The foot is in one of those fancy, tooled leather cowboy boots. The man the leg belongs to is in surgery having a nice stump fashioned by one of our surgeons.

"Seems the guy came around a blind corner on his motorcycle going about seventy, and ran into a minivan." *(Sound of a door opening and footsteps.)*

"The tech who tags and bags bodies for the morgue just came in. Hey Rich, what's up?"

"Nothing much. This the leg?"

"Yep, sorta looks like it don't you think?"

"How the hell am I supposed to toe tag this thing?"

"I don't know, Rich, but the one thing I do know for damned sure is that we're not taking off that boot."

"Oh come on Darcy, I've got to get the tag on it."

"Tag the boot."

"I don't think that'll fly with the people in charge."

"Tough. If you want to fish the foot out of that boot you go right ahead. Right now, I'm going to the back room for some coffee." (*Sound of a door opening.*) "Come and get me when you're done."

"Hey! Come back, Darcy. I'll make you a deal—If you write up the discharge papers, I'll—"

(*Darcy laughs.*) "If you think I'm going to write up discharge papers for a freaking *leg*, pal, you're nuts."

"Aw, come on."

(*In the background is the sound of squealing tires.*)

"I won't do it, Rich, so don't even—Oh shit! Hey! Somebody get a gurney out here STAT!" (*Sound of running, and tape is turned off.*)

"Well, I'm in my driveway. We got a kid who was having a serious asthma attack, and then after that, things got so crazy, I didn't have time to mess with the tape recorder.

"I'm exhausted, so I'll tie this up by saying that it's the pace of the ER that I love. That, and being able to take people from death's door and bring them back to the land of the living.

"And if the patient dies despite what we do, I like being able to put the survivors back together enough to function and get on with life.

"All of that has its own reward."

WANDA

"I fell into nursing because when you grow up in the back country of Alabama, there aren't a lot of other options for women. But once I was in it, I realized I got attached too easily to the patients and took all the emotional baggage home with me. It was like riding an emotional roller coaster every day.

"I switched to working ER when I discovered it's a great way to avoid attachments. It's always chaotic, so I don't have time to get attached. The more action the better—that way I don't have to stop and deal with each person on a personal level. Still, there are some situations where someone will just grab me and say, "I'm fixing to die. Please don't let me die." That never fails to get to me.

"Then there are the kids. When we lose a kid, it wastes me. I can barely bring myself to return for my next shift. Last summer we had a week where a child died every day in our ER—there were two drownings, a SIDS death, a bicycle vs. automobile death, and a ten-year-old boy who had been misdiagnosed by his pediatrician as a stress-triggered asthmatic, when in fact he was having a massive coronary due to a heart that was three-fourths the size of his chest.

"No debriefings were offered to the nurses who worked that week. Right after that that, they quit, one after the other. I just walked around angry. I was angry that we couldn't save those kids. I was angry that people were so stupid as to allow their children to go

unsupervised in a pool, or that they didn't have the common sense to teach their children basic bicycle safety, or know that there was something more wrong with their child than asthma.

"There is a status about being an ER nurse that puts you above other nurses. The patient's journey through the medical system often starts with the ER nurse. She's the one who calls the shots initially.

"The pace in an emergency room is a killer, but that's good— it doesn't give you a lot of time to feel anything.

"People are strange. The longer I work in ER, the stranger they get. Working ER really leaves me wondering how people can be so clueless."

This is one of those tasteless, black humor medical stories that the regular guy on the street would never understand, but medical people find funny.

We're in a big tourist town in the South, so we get a lot of travelers especially during the summer. One brutally hot July afternoon, an older couple came in. The husband said he'd played nine holes of golf that morning, and as he wasn't used to the extremes of our weather, had overextended himself. His chest pain started right around the fifth hole.

The cardiac bloods and EKG confirmed he was having a heart attack. Luckily, the guy had a first-rate insurance policy, so we did the whole cardiac shebang—TPA, nitroglycerine, lines, Lasix, morphine.

Understandably, his wife was frantic, terrified he might die and that she would be left stranded in a strange place by herself. A few hours after he was stabilized, we encouraged the wife to go back to the hotel and get some rest.

Five minutes after she left, she came running back into the ER holding a small bundle wrapped in a baby blanket and screaming bloody murder.

My first thought was that they must have left a grandchild in the car, so I grabbed the blanket and ran like hell, yelling for a pediatric code all the way to the trauma room.

As medical staff poured into the room, I lay the bundle down and opened the blanket. The poodle, left forgotten in the car, had died of heat stroke.

Blame it on the letdown of adrenaline, or maybe the heat had unbalanced our minds, but we all cracked up.

When we finally gained control of ourselves, someone managed to take the dog's owner to the meditation room, where he gave her the sad news.

Around here, Thanksgiving night is a guaranteed mass trauma night. Christmas, New Years, and the Fourth of July are nothing compared to Thanksgiving. Last Thanksgiving took the prize with one of those wrecks that everyone remembers forever.

It was around 9 p.m. that we got word from the sheriff's dispatcher that there'd been a bad wreck in which a passenger car swerved part way out of his lane on a sharp curve and hit a recreational vehicle head-on.

We were setting up the trauma rooms when the first ambulances arrived with the bodies from the RV—two grandparents, two parents, and six children—all dead. This was back in the days when trauma victims came directly to the hospital dead or alive. The bodies would then be laid out on gurneys next to each other until the doctor or the coroner could get to them.

The nurse who was taking care of the driver of the passenger car, was being unmercifully cruel to him. She'd refused the man the most basic of care, and called him a murderer to his face. At one point she pulled back the curtains so he had to look at the victims' bodies.

I ordered her out of the department and took over his care, but her poison had already started to work on him. The man was completely destroyed.

He told me he'd spent the day working on a building he was converting into a fishing equipment store, the dream of a lifetime come true.

On his way home, he took one of the downhill curves a little too fast and had gone over the centerline by a couple of feet. The oncoming RV was also a little over the line from his side. The two collided, and the RV went through the guardrails and over the edge.

The driver of the passenger car admitted he'd had a beer some eight hours earlier with his lunch, and was agonizing over the fact it may have impaired his judgment even though his blood alcohol level was negligible.

I recall thinking how easily any one of us could have been sitting in his place. How many nights had we gone out for a drink or two after work? How many times had I been in a hurry and taken a curve too fast, a tad over the line? I wanted to tell him this, but the look in his eyes made me keep my mouth shut. No rationalization was ever going to touch him, and no excuse would ever be enough.

It was about midday when a man ran in holding his son, a boy of about nine. As Dad told the story, the two of them had been out on their boat, fishing.

The boy had a terror of snakes, so the father, seeing this as a weakness in his son, decided to help him get over what he called a "sissy's fear."

A distance from shore, the dad reached into the water and pulled out a big old snake then proceeded to force it on his son.

The boy put up a fuss, begging his father not to make him touch it, but his daddy taunted him, and eventually forced the boy to hold the snake. Of course as soon as the kid had the thing in his hand, the snake bit him.

The boy came in to us sicker than hell with his arm swollen to three times its normal size. As fate would have it, we were fortunate enough to have a doctor on staff who was one of America's foremost experts on poisonous snakes, so the child was in good hands.

Meanwhile, out in the waiting room, the father still had the snake in his tackle box for identification. I grew up in the backcountry, so I know snakes better than most women, and I know how to handle them with respect. The minute he opened his tackle box, I knew it was a cottonmouth, one of the most venomous snakes around.

I know it wasn't right, but I was so hopping mad, I couldn't help myself. I still can't believe I didn't lose my job over it, but at the time I don't think I would have cared if I had.

I yanked that tackle box right out of that man's hands and opened it up wide. I then chased that son-of-a-bitch around the room yelling, "Here! Stick your hand in here big guy! Come on, bully-boy, let's see if you do as well as your little boy."

He looked at me like I was crazy, but I'll tell you, that bully sure did run!

PETER ALLAR
St. Vincent's Hospital, ER nurse
Department Nurse Educator
New York City resident

"My first career was in graphic arts, publishing and printing—jobs I found completely unsatisfying. Around that time, my mother died from breast cancer. The care she had received from her doctors and nurses was so harsh and insensitive, that it propelled me to volunteer at hospices in Virginia Beach and Norfolk, Virginia, where I cared for people who were dying. In 1985 I moved from Virginia Beach to New York City and shortly after that, I volunteered to work with AIDS patients for the Gay Men's Health Crisis organization. Finally, on the prodding of friends, I enrolled in St. Vincent's nursing school.

"There is nothing better than ER nursing. We have the reputation of being rough. We save lives but we color outside the lines. We're independent and we tiptoe around the Rules of Nursing."

September 11, 2001
New York City

I was scheduled to work with two ER orientees that day. One was a patient care technician and the other was an RN who had not worked in ER before. I'd just placed them with preceptors in the ER and was standing by the nursing station talking to one of the other nurses, when one of our doctors, Craig Tenenbaum, left to teach a Pediatric Advanced Life Support class down on Seventh Avenue. He couldn't have been gone three minutes when he ran back into the ER and announced, "A plane just hit the World Trade Center!"

We didn't comprehend at first, and said, "Yeah, sure, Craig. You're just tired. You need to go home and get some sleep."

He was insistent. "No, no!" he said. "You don't understand. A plane really did just hit the World Trade Center."

We realized then that he wasn't kidding. At that point I thought maybe it was a small, single engine plane and we might get a few patients, because how could a larger plane crash into such a large building, right? But Craig said, "No, it was a commercial airliner. A seven-sixty-seven. I watched it fly into the building."

It was such a preposterous idea, that we thought we were having a surprise disaster drill and that Craig was part of the drill. It was the expression on his face that convinced us that he wasn't acting. As soon as I realized that he was serious, we focused on what had to be done and got busy.

The hospital called a Code Three on the overhead system, which meant an external disaster, something we'd not had since the first World Trade Center bombing a decade earlier. We'd had a disaster drill a couple of months before, using a strategy we'd developed.

I gathered my two orientees and told them what was about to happen was really going to be something and that they were about to be baptized into the ER by fire. I told them to get organized, focus on the important things, follow directions, and above all, not to panic.

We transferred the existing ER patients to several other open areas of the hospital so that the ER was completely cleared. At the same time, we mobilized all the nurse managers and float nurses to their assigned areas. It was like that calm before the storm because the magnitude of what was going to happen didn't register with anybody at that point.

Most of us were working at St. Vincent's when the World Trade Center got hit the first time, so we were thinking in terms of smoke inhalation and burns.

I was assigned to triage where nurses focus on the basic factors: Is the patient breathing? Are they stable or unstable?

It took a while for the first patient to show up, but when they did come, they came in groups—six patients or more per ambulance drop off. Most of those first patients were extremely critical, some with terrible burns that left their skin completely blackened. There was one person I later found out was a fireman, who came in with CPR in progress, in cardiac arrest.

Those first cases flashed right by us to Unit Five, critical care. It was so fast. I'd glance up and see a stretcher go by with someone on it who had no skin or hair and was being ventilated with an Ambu bag.

One of the first patients was an older woman who'd been badly burned to the extent that her skin was like a black crust that fell off onto the floor. We put in an IV and started resuscitation fluids and pain meds then tried to cut off as much of her clothing as possible, except it had melted into her skin. That was hard to see.

The first real inkling I had of the magnitude of the devastation was when the paramedics started saying that we wouldn't believe what was going on down there. They told us there were so many victims that they were being directed to leave some of them behind. What that meant was that some of the victims were so critically injured, they were being left to die at the scene.

That was very troubling to the paramedics and EMTs, and some of them weren't the same after that. One paramedic I was close to suffered terrible depression and PTSD and couldn't return to work. He felt that he had failed to rescue people, which was his call to duty.

Then the rescue workers started telling us that bodies were flying through the air, landing right in front of them. One body fell on a firefighter and killed him.

They were stepping over body parts, heads, arms and legs, to get to the people they could save. I watched their faces as they told us this, and realized that it was all horrifically true.

A bit later, people started running in to tell us that a second plane had hit the other tower. Afterward, we were told that the buildings had collapsed. I couldn't stop what I was doing, but I remember thinking, *The buildings collapsed? What does that mean?* I couldn't even visualize it. While the entire world was watching what was happening on the TV, we were very much cocooned inside the Emergency Department. We had no idea of the enormity of the disaster unfolding less than a mile away.

Staying calm was the main problem—everyone was really nervous. When you see the cops and the EMS people getting nervous, it makes everyone nervous.

When people came in and said that the Pentagon had been hit, I remember saying to Nancy Issing that our whole world had just changed forever. At the time I was being dramatic, but it ended up being a true statement.

I don't think Nancy could handle hearing it said aloud, because she just looked at me and said, "Shut up Peter and keep working."

The one patient who stays with me was a fireman, a big, strapping young guy who was in absolute shock. When he came in, his face was totally blank—no emotion at all. He told one of the nurses that he and his partner were running out of the building as it started to collapse. His partner suddenly went limp and started to fall, so he blindly grabbed him and was running with him in his arms when he realized that his partner had been decapitated. I was listening to this man talk, but I was unable to fully grasp what he was saying.

Right after that we had a cop come in looking for his partner, and then all these paramedics came in right behind him, looking for the rest of their crews. It was absolutely crushing. I felt so guilty because everyone I knew was alive and safe.

When the patients stopped coming, I thought at first that they were all buried and the rescue workers would start digging them out soon. So we remained prepared for them.

3 p.m.

I ran home to change my clothes. There were dozens of messages on my machine from people I knew who were calling to say how proud they were of what we were doing and that they loved me.

When I got back to the hospital there were hundreds of people lined up all along the sidewalk across the street watching what was happening. People were stopping me in the street asking, "What can we do to help? Where can we donate blood? What do you guys need?"

The local Starbucks on Greenwich Avenue kept bringing us fresh coffee, and the old Italian women from the neighborhood brought in pans of baked ziti and lasagna.

The other group of people that began coming in were the relatives and loved ones searching for their friends and family. This was the beginning of the "Have You Seen" posters. That was heartbreaking because I realized there was no chance that their loved ones were alive. But they had hope that somehow their loved one was just missing, misidentified, or stuck somewhere in a corner.

12 a.m.

By about midnight there were no more patients, so I went home to sleep. I turned on the TV and watched the whole thing for the first time. I was just overwhelmed. I'm not a person who cries, but I felt like the world had changed, which on that day it did.

It was the first time I saw the World Trade Center towers collapse. It seemed impossible, but there it was.

September 12, 2001
5 a.m.

I went back to the hospital because I couldn't sleep. There were all these rumors about people being pulled out. We waited all day, but they never came.

September 14, 2001

It rained hard and all I could think was that if there were still people down there alive, they were being rained on and would be cold and wet. We knew there was no hope for them.

It was at this point that we began caring for the rescue workers who were working down at the pit. Many of them had respiratory problems requiring nebulizer therapy. Years from now we will know just how environmentally toxic that situation was.

September 17, 2001

That awful smell started coming from Ground Zero. Nobody had to ask what it was—you knew what it was. I lived not far from Ground Zero and for months there was a fine gray ash that would creep in and collect on my windowsills. When I would clean, I'd wonder, *Am I wiping up people?*

To see those desperate faces coming in at all hours of the day and night looking for their loved ones? Oh it was so sad, I can't tell you. They'd come with flyers and photographs and end up going from hospital to hospital.

I realized the people they were looking for were probably dead and they knew it too, but just couldn't admit it to themselves. They'd sit there while you went through the lists, then they'd beg you to go through it again.

And the calls? There were hundreds of calls from people looking for loved ones. We didn't want to tell them there was no hope, so we'd just say they weren't here and to call again or go to the other hospitals.

Everywhere you went in the city were hung pictures of the missing. I found myself identifying with two photos of a young lady and young man. Under the one photo, the boy's mother had written, "This is my son. If you see him, please call me."

I see those two faces in my mind knowing they will never be found—they follow me everywhere I go.

February 2002

I've been having horrendous dreams about the planes hitting and the buildings exploding. I recently had a dream of NYU being blown up.

I still feel guilty for not going down to Ground Zero and helping someone out of the rubble. I should have just gone down there right away. The real heroes were the people who were down there.

Me? I'm not a hero—I was in a safe place doing what I always do, but on a larger scale that day. I didn't put my life in jeopardy like they did.

I think it's going to happen again, and when it does, we'll do a great job of overcoming it. I think as a group, the ER nurses were heroes because we came together and kept ourselves and everybody else together. People were so willing to do whatever it took. I'm just glad I could be a part of it.

December 2014

My two most vivid memories of 9/11 are actually from the weekend before the event. A large group of us from the ER had taken a bus trip down to Atlantic City for the day. Just before we left, I went into the Starbucks across the street from the hospital to get coffee for the trip. Standing in line in front of me was Graydon Carter, editor-in-chief of *Vanity Fair*. He was conversing with another man and I overheard him say, "There has never been a better time to be in New York."

All these years later that statement has stuck with me because it was so true—New York was idyllic at that moment in time. Yet, only a few days later, that "no better time" was violently taken away.

The second memory was related to our return trip. It was dusk, and as we rode down the roadway leading to the Holland Tunnel, the World Trade Center came into view, the setting sun striking it so that the buildings were luminous. It was so beautiful. It made for a perfect last picture of the landmark since I never saw the WTC again except as smoldering wreckage.

I visited the 9/11 memorial and museum this fall. I hated the memorial. It was the typically over-thought governmental memorial site—sterile, cold, and impersonal. I wish they had just left the two holes as they were, and allowed vegetation to fill it in. Life renewed.

The museum was another story. I went by myself but I wish I had brought someone with me because it is a place to share memories and feelings. The collection of pieces connected to humans—a crushed ambulance, a destroyed fire truck—seeing these things was sobering.

However, it was the Survivor's Staircase that made the biggest impact on me. The stairs were originally part of two outdoor flights that connected Vesey Street to the World Trade Center's Tobin Plaza. On 9/11, these very same stairs served as an escape route for hundreds of evacuees from 5 World Trade Center to the street. The stairs themselves are crumbled, the blood stains still visible. Most of the stairs had been destroyed, but this one piece had made it through. I used to climb those stairs and stare up at the two massive buildings, contemplating things.

Now, St. Vincent's staff is dispersed, and St. Vincent's itself is gone, torn down in order to build multi-million dollar condos. But those of us who worked there on that clear blue morning, can always look back on how we were a dynamic team on America's darkest day.

MAGGIE

"Let me put it to you straight—I love the adrenaline rush of the ER. I've worked trauma centers in LA, Tampa, and Boston for sixteen years and I'm still hooked on that rush. It was emergency work that brought me into nursing, not vice versa.

"I like making order out of chaos. On my own, I can take a totally messed up human being and within a matter of minutes have them settled down, stabilized, packaged up and on their way out the door whistling Dixie.

"I started out as a paralegal and then became an EMT working weekends at big racecar events. I've been an adrenaline junkie ever since. In the way that people have to pay initiation dues to join a club, I had to work ICU before I could go to ER. It was a near worthless experience except I finally figured out why ICU and ER nurses have such a hostile relationship. It's simple, really. The ICU nurses are single task oriented; the ER nurses are process oriented.

"ICU nurses are into babysitting the doctors. (She mimics a high, whiny voice.) 'Oh we can't possibly call Dr. so-and-so because he'll get angry with me.' That sort of co-dependent, passivity horseshit would make an ER nurse insane inside of twenty seconds.

"ICU nurses believe they are the organized, clean folks, and that ER nurses are messy chaos freaks. Anal-retentive vs. free

spirits in the big picture. It isn't quite that way. ER nurses are fast and thorough—ICU nurses are slow and thorough.

"Actually, what it boils down to is that nurses piss on whoever is bringing them the work. ER nurses piss on paramedics, ICU and everybody else who receive patients from us, piss on the ER nurses. But it's like, hey get over it, this is what we do.

"At one time I worked in an ER in a very toxic hospital that I dubbed Satan's Medical Center. I was so traumatized after my shifts there that I would have to debrief with my husband every night. When he couldn't stand to hear it anymore, I debriefed with my best friend until the day I told her about the man who came in complaining about the leg of lamb stuck up his ass and no clue as to how it got there—and she didn't laugh. I just remember her looking at me with this horrified expression while I roared with laughter.

"I've had to develop other ways to deal with what I see every day, so I've gone a little tough around the edges. I'm at the point now where a situation has to be a major shrieker for me to even give it a second thought.

"But, really, considering what I see every day, I'm amazed that there are still things that get to me."

Satan's Medical Center, a Catholic-run institution, was an evil, accursed place to be introduced into ER nursing. It was baptism by the fires of Hell itself. It was a place of such an uncaring and malicious nature, that any one of us could have intentionally killed a patient and no one would have noticed, much less cared. The apathetic atmosphere contaminated every situation that spun through those doors.

Every day I worked at Satan's was frustrating, but the most heinous situation that I have ever witnessed and been made a part of, involved a man who slid his motorcycle under the front of a big rig.

On their way to the burn center with this man, the ambulance crew somehow got lost and ended up at our facility. I saw the medical transport vehicle pull into the ambulance bay and thought it was weird, considering no one had radioed us about a medical transport.

The vehicle screeched to a stop and the driver literally jumped out of the cab running and waving her arms. When she saw me, she took hold of my scrub top and began pulling me toward the ambulance.

"You've got to help this guy!" she yelled, "Christ Almighty, get the morphine! Give him something to make him stop screaming!"

The woman was hysterical, and that translated in my mind that she had to be a rookie. I took her by the shoulders and made her look at me. "I don't know what you're talking about. Take a deep breath and make sense."

"Twenty-two-year-old guy," she gasped, pointing at the ambulance with trembling hands. "Slid his motorcycle under the front end of a semi. The bike exploded. He's got third degree burns everywhere. We were told to get him to C— Burn Center. I took the wrong exit and got lost. Yours was the first hospital I saw."

She moved quickly to the rig's back doors. "He's been screaming since we left. He needs morphine. We don't carry it. You've got to give him something or he's going to—"

She flung open the doors, and the rest of her words were drowned out by shrieking, the likes of which I'd never heard before or since. I took one look at the man and went into an adrenaline charged panic.

What lay on the stretcher more resembled a piece of meat that someone had left too long on the barbecue, than a human being. His eyelids had been burned away, so there were these two naked, terror-filled eyeballs staring right at me. If he had not been screaming, I would not have believed he could still be alive.

I took off like a madwoman back into the ER yelling for the ER doc du jour, Dr. S. He stuck his head out of an exam room and glowered at me.

"Give me an order for ten of morphine," I shouted as I jogged toward the narcotics lockbox. "We've got a man en route to the burn center with third degree burns over seventy percent of his body. They don't have any MS on their rig. How about five milligrams intravenously, provided I can find a vein, and then another five in two minutes?"

Dr. S sucked in his cheeks and his eyes narrowed to slits. "I'm not giving orders for anything," he said coolly. "I don't know this person from Adam."

My mouth fell open and I stared in disbelief. "Can't you hear that man screaming out there? Let's give him some MS and let them get him to the burn center. We can deal with the legal formalities later."

"I've got nothing to do with this patient. He's not ours." And then, he closed the door.

I was stunned. I imagined that the screaming man in the rig was my husband or my son, and, in an unprecedented move, I flung open the door he'd just closed and demanded that he come into the hall. There, in front of God and everyone, I begged like a child.

Instead of softening, Dr. S became enraged, going from zero to a hundred in two seconds. "I'll see this patient," he said in a barely controlled voice, "When you admit him like a regular ER patient."

"But he's not a regular patient. He's a burn patient on his way to a burn center. Let's break with regulations and policies just this once. A little morphine and he'll be on his way. I'll take care of the incident reports later."

A volley of the man's screams punctuated my point, and for a minute, Dr. S seemed to reconsider.

"He's a regular patient until I've evaluated him," he said. "I won't give an order for morphine until after I've seen him."

All the way to the rig, I cursed the arrogant son of a suffering bitch, praying that someday he would burn in the hottest part of Hell.

Meanwhile, the man's shrieks had escalated. Not that he had any real chance at survival—he was a crispy critter and he was going to die in the next one to twelve hours no matter what we did.

After I got the guy into trauma, I drew up a syringe of morphine while Dr. S took his own bloody sweet Jesus time about seeing him. First he stopped to check something on one of the discharge charts, and then he checked on a patient with a sore throat.

A long agonized shriek came from the trauma room and echoed down the hall as Dr. S ambled to the drinking fountain for a sip of water. He shuffled back to the chart rack and randomly perused another chart.

I went into what I call the Red Zone, a condition of the temper from which there is no return. My own skin crawling with sympathetic pain, I shoved the chart into Dr. S's hands and got up in his bloated, miserable face.

"That man in there is suffering the agonies of Hell while you're out here lollygagging around with your thumb stuck up your ass. He needs morphine and fluids now or we're going to have a code on our hands."

Dr. S picked up a chart on a patient who'd come in with a sprained ankle. "I've already told you that I'd see that patient when it's his turn."

My brain twisted around on itself and for a second or two I truly believed I was in the presence of pure evil; a reincarnate Dr. Josef Mengele.

I backed away a little fearful, unable to grasp the extent of his inhuman brutality. How anyone could so casually ignore the tormented screams of another human being was beyond me.

Was it to defy us, the female underlings? Or, was it to let all know that he was in charge and did not have to do what he jolly well didn't want to?

I think that if a weapon had suddenly materialized in my hand, I would have used it on this evil asshole without a second thought.

"I'm giving the patient five milligrams of morphine now," I said, making my way to the trauma room. "I cannot allow a human being to suffer this way."

He blocked my way. "You give that man morphine without a physician's order and I'll have your license." The vein in his forehead was engorged and throbbing. "You'll never practice nursing again."

"I don't care," I said, stepping around him. "I refuse to let this man die in torment. It's not humane."

He wrapped his hand around the upper part of my arm and jerked me back like a rag doll.

The clerk, a sweet girl who had not yet been hardened by her work environment, shot out of her chair and rushed over to us. "Hey, cool it guys," she whispered. "Dispatch called the guy's mom. She's right behind you watching all three rings of this circus."

Dr. S and I turned at the same time. In the alcove next to the water fountain sat a distraught looking woman hunched at the shoulders. She was staring at the physician with intense hatred in her eyes.

I shuddered to think she had witnessed this monster parading as a physician, drag his feet while her son screamed in unimaginable agony.

Dr. S's insolent expression at once dissolved into something between fear and contempt.

"Phew," I said just loud enough for him to hear, "Can't you just smell that malpractice suit brewing?"

Dr. S pushed me out of the way and, dialing up his stock expression of grave concern, slithered over to the woman. Committing acts of verbal bowing, scraping and downright lying, he assured the woman her son was receiving the best care that could be provided.

I found it ironic that this last lie was accompanied by the sound of her son's agonized screams.

She listened to his bullshit, and even nodded a few times as though she fully understood, then she looked him full in the eyes and asked what kind of a blind and deaf fool he thought she was. Then, as if Betty Davis and Joan Crawford were cheering her on, she slapped him hard across the face.

I medicated the patient with as much morphine as I dared pump into him and sent him on his way. I caught up with his mother in the parking lot and handed her a paper on which I'd written Dr. S's name, the phone number for the hospital's administrative offices, and the name and number of an honest malpractice attorney.

Of course Dr. S never did sign the morphine order, but by the time the administrative police found the discrepancy, I was long gone.

People ask me about whether or not I see miracles in the ER. I suppose the answer is yes, but there is usually a pretty good explanation behind every ER miracle.

Take for instance, the young Latino who'd just landed his first good paying job with a roofing company. On his first day of work, within the first hour, he fell forty feet through a skylight and landed on his head, sustaining significant head injuries.

When he came into ER, he was unstable and unresponsive except for some weak movement in one hand. When we sent him up to ICU, we were pretty certain he wouldn't survive.

About two weeks later I was scheduled to work in ICU and, since no one likes taking care of a brain dead corpse, the kid was assigned to me.

While I was doing my initial neuro assessment, I noticed the fingers of his "good" hand seemed to be moving in a purposeful way, as if he were tapping out a rhythm. On top of that, I was pretty sure he was making attempts to assist the ventilator with his own breaths.

When the internist came in, he stuck his head in the patient's room, and shouted a few commands from the door: Open your eyes, move your left hand, lift your leg, smile if you can understand what I'm saying.

Nada. Not a twitch. The patient was as unresponsive as a rock.

The doctor went out to the nurses' station to write his progress notes. I read over his shoulder that he believed the kid's prognosis was zilch. His recommendation? Start weaning him off life support and let him die.

"Actually," I said, as the doctor was signing off his notes, "The patient is moving his right hand with purpose, and he's making attempts to breathe. I'm not sure you can interpret that as circling the drain."

The doc reacted to my comment in the same way most doctors respond to nurses' notes, which is to say, not at all.

My patient's mother came in an hour later. Her English was poor, but she understood well enough when I told her that unless her son showed some sign that proved his brain was working, it would not go well for him.

She didn't have to think long. Without a moment's hesitation, she marched into her son's room barking urgent sounding Spanish. Before she finished her first volley of commands, his eyes flew open and he began hitting the siderail with one hand.

I studied his face, noting that his mouth was working ever so slightly. I was sure that he was trying to talk around the endotracheal tube.

An hour later, the neurologist showed up and, to his credit, actually went inside the patient's room. Wearing his best mournful expression, he leaned against the bedrails and stared at his patient. He whispered a few commands in the same tone one might pray over a close relative's grave, then returned to the desk and wrote orders that concurred with the internist's—discontinue all life support and let the kid die.

"But the boy responds to verbal stimuli," I argued.

The neurologist frowned, checked the internist's note again, then looked at me over the tops of his bifocals. "Well, he doesn't have much of a brain left so I doubt that very much."

I pulled the pen out of his hand. "Listen," I said, "This kid has reflexes and—"

The neurologist rolled his eyes. "You're seeing autonomic reflexes, like a chicken after its head is cut off." He flashed me a tight smile and took back his pen.

"Tell you what," I said. "Go in there and explain to his mother that you're losing hope and that it might be time to remove life support. Then ask her to give him some commands."

He considered for a moment. Then, just to let me know how much my request was putting him out, he heaved an "I-don't-know-why-I-let-you-nurses-talk-me-into-this-nonsense" sigh, and gave it a go.

Mom repeated whatever it was she'd said earlier, only this time in an even harsher tone, and again, the kid's eyes flew open and he jiggled the siderails, as if he were trying to escape.

The doc blinked, nodded to the mother, and went to the desk to call the internist and explain why they weren't going to pull the kid off life support.

Six months later, the boy and his mother walked into ICU to thank us for saving his life. I hadn't been able to stop thinking about what had happened that day, so I asked the mother what she'd said to her son that made him have such an immediate strong reaction.

Laughing, she said, "I told him that unless he showed the doctor he could open his eyes and move around a little, they were going to cut off his penis!"

Lest anyone think I'm a doctor hater, let me assure you that I am not—I am only a hater of incompetence and laziness in any healthcare professional. Sometime during my second year at Satan's, a young heroin addict wandered out onto the freeway and was hit by multiple cars. His airway was shot and he was coughing up blood and tissue all over everybody. He was, as they say in the ER, a train wreck racing for the station.

This was right in the beginning of AIDS and universal blood precautions, so I didn't have goggles or gloves on, and I was getting this man's blood in my eyes, my face, up my nose. It was a total blood bath.

I was trying to stabilize the man's neck when Dr. X told me to take the patient the CT scanner.

"No way," I said. "This dude is going to code in the scanner. I won't take him unless you go with me."

"It's okay," Dr. X says, "You go ahead and I'll be right there."

Stamp an "S" for Sucker on my forehead, because I took the guy to the scanner by myself. Sure enough, within five minutes after we got his head situated inside the doughnut hole, he codes and it's just the scanner tech and me.

We called six times for a code and not one person responded. I was doing CPR when one of the nurses stuck her head in the door, saw what was happening and did an about-face and left. A few minutes later a regular ER doc meandered over and ran a code for all of two minutes before she pronounced the guy.

I wrote an incident report on both Dr. X, who never did show, and the nurse who saw what was happening and ran. I personally handed the report to Sister B, the head of ER Quality Assurance along with a cover letter explaining why these folks needed counseling. I went on for pages about how we needed to protect the patients from sloppy and negligent care, and yadda, yadda.

As it happened, a week after I gave the report to Sister B, she dropped dead and one of the ER nurses was assigned to clean out her desk. In the bottom drawer, under two boxes of Kleenex, he found all the incident reports the ER nurses had written over the last three years regarding the various fatal or near-fatal mistakes made by incompetent medical personnel.

There were over three hundred unprocessed reports detailing all the corrupt and inhumane acts perpetrated on the unsuspecting patients, and she'd just shoved them into the bottom of her desk.

One of the downsides for people who work in the ER for too long is that they become jaded. Those of us who manage to maintain some level of compassion for long stretches of time are far and few between.

The first of the two cases that finally drove me out of Satan's Medical Center was an auto accident in which a drunk going fifty-five miles an hour broadsided another car.

In the car hit were a mother, father and a three-year-old girl strapped into her car seat. The impact was so great, that it sheared the child's safety seat literally in half.

The dad was mostly unhurt because he was opposite the side of impact, but the little girl had severe head injuries and basically came in brain dead. The mom received a deep laceration that extended from her hip to her knee. Following the Life Is Unfair Law, the driver of the other car didn't get a scratch.

The father was in emotional shock, walking around dazed, unable to talk to anyone, including the mother. The mother was hysterical, but couldn't do anything because she was so badly injured.

Dr. R, a big bear of a man at six-feet-five and three hundred pounds, was up to his armpits trying to resuscitate the little girl, but no one could ignore the fact that the entire time he worked on her, he was crying. I don't mean just tears running down his face; he was outright sobbing.

I kept patting him on the back, saying, "It's okay Dr. R, you're doing great. Hang in there, Dr. R, it's going to be okay."

We managed to stabilize the child long enough for the grandmother to come in to say good-bye. I have a vivid memory of her rocking that baby in her arms, looking at the ceiling and praying, "Dear God, take me instead. Oh God please take me now and let this child live."

At that, we all lost it. I just—I didn't—I'm sorry—(*The tape is paused.*) I didn't realize until after the child had been transferred to wherever they brought her to die that no one in that family received any counseling from our so-called social services. The priest who was on for social services didn't want his dinner interrupted, and the social worker had been cut back to three days a week.

The next shift came in while Dr. R and I were cleaning up the room. Both of us were still sobbing, and nobody else was doing much talking either.

The oncoming charge nurse waited until Dr. R left the unit then came at me like an enraged bull. "Get it together," she yelled, shaking her finger in my face. "You're an ER nurse. This kind of sentimental weakness has no place in this department. If you're going to breakdown every time you get a pediatric trauma, you need to get the hell out!"

I lost it completely. "And *you* shouldn't be a nurse if you can't be human! Sentimental weakness? If by that you mean human compassion, this ER needs all the sentimental weakness it can get!"

The next day I ran into Dr. R. and got him talking about what had happened. It turns out that he and his wife had lost a baby to SIDS eight months before and he'd not been able to grieve because he thought he had to be strong for his wife.

For all that time, he'd been stuffing that pain down inside himself. The moment he saw that little girl, all his sorrow and the suffering came to the surface.

It works like that with ER folks—sometimes a particular patient just gets to you and rips your heart out.

The case that finally caused me to resign from Satan's was a horror of another type. The incident I'm talking about took place fairly early in the day, after report had been given, but before the barrage of commuter traffic accidents had begun.

I'd just finished checking the crash cart when a woman who was obviously upset ran up to the ER clerk and began frantically pointing toward the parking lot at the rear of the hospital.

Thinking she was reporting a parking lot fender bender, I started to turn away, but the ER clerk turned pale and bolted out of her chair.

ER clerks have seen and heard it all, so I knew whatever the problem was, it had to be something especially heinous in the world of Satan's horrors.

The clerk dragged the woman over to me and instructed her to repeat her complaint.

"He's out in the parking lot, in front of everybody, taking photographs of a dead baby," the woman said, her voice breaking. "You've got to stop him!"

I looked the woman over carefully. She didn't look like a psycho. "I don't understand what you mean," I said.

"I'm telling you there's is a policeman out there who is taking pictures of a dead infant. A crowd has gathered and is watching him. It's unspeakable. It shouldn't be allowed!"

I had to admit that she seemed certain of her facts, but then I remembered that the county health fair was scheduled for the upcoming weekend. I was sure that what the woman had witnessed was one of our paramedics practicing on Resusci Baby—one of the lifelike dummies used when teaching pediatric CPR. It was probably a paramedic giving a community service demonstration and the local newspaper was taking photos to advertise the fair.

It being a slow morning, I could spare the time to explain this to the woman and walk with her to the parking lot. I would then ask the paramedics to make sure people knew Resusci Baby was only a practice dummy.

About sixty feet away, I saw a sheriff's deputy aiming a flash camera at the ground. Even with his back to me, I could see from the way he moved that he was comfortable with what he was doing. Just as the woman said, a small crowd had gathered around him to watch.

Through the picket fence of people's legs, I made out something small and white in the center of a blue tarp spread out on the ground. I squinted. It didn't look like Resusci Baby. An image of a bloated white piglet briefly crossed my mind.

I looked around for the paramedics, and when I didn't see them, I told the woman to stay where she was and began to walk faster.

The first thing I noticed when I reached the edge of the crowd was the silence. No one was talking. The next thing I saw was the expressions on people's faces. Some had covered their mouths, a few grimaced in disgust, a few were crying. All of them looked horrified.

I pushed my way through to the deputy, but by the time I got to him, he was throwing the sides of the tarp over whatever it was he'd been photographing.

The deputy couldn't have been any more than twenty-two. His hair was buzz cut so close to his scalp, he looked like a new boot camp recruit. He picked up the tarp with one hand and slung it into the open trunk of the patrol car like a sack of dirty laundry. Behind me, I heard low murmurs as the crowd disbursed.

"Excuse me," I said. "What were you photographing?"

He eyed my uniform with a look of suspicion, but when he realized I was a nurse, he must have assumed it would be okay to share the details.

"A dead infant," he answered as casually as he would have said, "A pile of dead leaves."

"Some white trash teenager down in W—ville delivered at home and threw the kid in a dumpster. The garbage men found it a couple of hours ago and brought it here. I was told to pick it up, bring it to the county morgue and take photos."

I was almost too stunned to speak—almost.

"What kind of insensitive, mindless asshole lays out a dead infant in the middle of a public parking for all to see while he photographs it?"

Instead of answering the question, the cop went apeshit and threatened to arrest me for interfering with the process of the law. When he got into the cruiser, I had a feeling that wouldn't be the end of it.

It wasn't. The deputy reported me to the hospital administration and within the hour I found myself in front of the director of nurses being formally charged with inappropriate behavior.

I tried to make her understand by carefully explaining what had taken place in the parking lot, but she refused to hear it. I was placed on six-months probation.

The next day, I turned in my resignation and that was the end of my days in Hell at Satan's House of Half-assed Medicine.

CLEO

"I work part-time in the ER, and part-time in ICU. I have tried to be a positive bridge over those troubled and murky waters between the two units. To say it is a difficult task is a major understatement."

It wasn't Halloween, the circus wasn't in town, and there weren't any weird parades going on. For these reasons, I couldn't come up with any excuse for the lineup of patients in our ER that night.

Gurney #1, a finger laceration, was a fifty-six-year-old man who wore a large purple top hat, like the one worn by the Mad Hatter. He refused to take it off, stating that he wore it everywhere he went. In fact, he said that the only time he ever took it off was to change into a black top hat for formal occasions.

Gurney #2, a rusty nail puncture, was a ninety-five-year-old World War I vet, dressed up in his old uniform and playing his harmonica non-stop.

Gurney #3, infected whip wounds, was a couple dressed in spiked dog collars, black leather and red and blue spiked hair.

Gurney #4, a bead stuck in nasal passage, was a three-year-old girl wearing iridescent angel wings and a glittering halo.

The ER doc coming on duty walked into the room took a long look at the lineup, and then at me. "What? No dancing midgets?"

I was still laughing when Bess, my nurse partner in crime and best friend, asked me to help with her alcoholic patient who was going into DTs (delirium tremens). The patient was a long time ER frequent flyer we'd nicknamed Wild Bill Wacko.

Wild Bill was only thirty-eight but looked like he'd been rode hard and put away wet a hundred years ago. Skinny and pale, his hair was in a messy braid down his back, and his beard was so long, he kept it tucked into his pants. He said he wore it that way to keep it from "interfering."

Wild Bill had a lot of alcohol onboard. As if that wasn't enough, he'd added a bottle of Nyquil and some sterno. As far as we could tell, his hallucinations involved a rodeo and a bus. Screams of, "Whoa Nellie! Somebody rope that bull," and, "Get me off this bus, you old sidewinder. Thar's the saloon!" rang throughout the ER.

This was regardless of the fact that over the preceding sixty minutes, Bess had given him enough lorazepam, an antianxiety agent, to kill the horse he was riding. On top of that, he'd been given Haldol, an antipsychotic medication.

The fact that he wasn't intubated, had Bess and me a little nervous to say the least. I kept waiting for him to crash, or, in his words, "fall out of the damned saddle."

ICU called to ask if we could transfer him to a regular electric hospital bed and hold him until they could make room for him upstairs. About thirty minutes after we'd gotten him into an electric bed, Wild Bill suddenly stopped yelling. Sixty seconds of silence elapsed when my gut told me something was hinkey.

I went flying into the exam room only to find that he'd managed to slip out of his hand restraints and was ripping out his intravenous lines. Blood was everywhere. It looked like a steer—or perhaps his horse—had been slaughtered.

Bess and I had just managed to get one of his hands restrained, when he yelled, "Yippee ki-yay! Let 'er rip Jenny!" and peed all over the bed. It was a fountainous amount of pee, one of those full-stream urinations that go on forever.

We were in the middle of doing some flood control, when an electrical burning smell filled the room. I started sniffing like mad, frantically trying to locate the source of the smell, when Wild Bill let loose with renewed whooping.

Before our eyes, the bed began to buck. Sparks flying, smoke pouring from underneath, the shorted out steel bronco moved across the floor.

Holding onto the sheets, Wild Bill Wacko sat bolt upright and waved an imaginary Stetson over his head. "Hee haw," he screamed. "Hang on little doggies!"

I turned around to see Bess in the corner, laughing so hard she couldn't stand up.

The bed continued to buck toward the door as Wild Bill put his invisible hat back on and made motions as if he was smoking a joint.

Looking back over his shoulder, eyes half-mast, he smiled broadly, showing off his lack of teeth. "Say, you gals want to smoke some of this here weed? It's gotta be the best damned shit I ever lit up!"

That did it. I barely managed to pull the plug on the bed before I collapsed next to Bess.

One of our third year residents entered the room and took in the scene. "How the hell did I get in Psych?" he said and walked out.

That knocked us right back into wheezing mode.

BOB DEMBICKI
Director, Cornell Burn Unit, NYC
New York City resident

"I don't know exactly why I became a nurse except for the fact that when I was fifteen I was a patient and I admired the nurses for what they did and the way they did it. Whatever it was, it drove me, because I was a nurse by the time I was nineteen.

"There is a huge range of disciplines in burn nursing because the patient has such a multitude of needs. We have to think of everything from making sure the environment is perfectly sterile, to the dietary and psychological needs of each individual.

"In short, burns are an entirely different world of nursing."

September 11, 2001
New York City

Living in the city of New York, we, as residents, think often about terrorism. We have more cultural diversity here than anywhere in the world. I live down the street from the United Nations, and because this is the heartbeat of the world, I think the possibility of terrorist attacks is always in the back of people's minds.

That day, we were having a critical care open house for nurses—trying to get them interested in working here.

I was in the conference room showing people around, when someone came by and said that a plane had just crashed into the World Trade Center. I thought that maybe a small commuter plane crashed into a corner of the building and we might get a few burn victims.

When I called upstairs to get people ready for the patients, I was told that the "small plane" was in fact a jumbo jet. When the second tower was hit, I think everyone thought we were under terrorist attack.

Unfortunately, the unit was unusually full already. We had six kids and thirty some-odd other patients. All I could think was, *Oh my god, at least fifty thousand people work in those buildings at any given time. How are we going to handle this?*

Between 9 and 9:30, I began the process of moving people out of our Burn ICU. Within twenty minutes we had eight beds vacated, stocked, cleaned ceiling to floor and ready to take patients. It was a blur to me at the time, but when I look back on it, I wondered how the hell we managed to do that. However we did it, it was just in time, because the victims started rolling in at 9:30.

Within fifteen minutes we got eight patients who had sixty to a hundred percent burns from jet fuel. Somewhere in the midst of that hell, we received word that the towers had fallen. That was the most devastating news, because those buildings were huge, and we knew that anyone who didn't get out before they collapsed, wasn't going to get out. There was no way anyone could survive under that many tons of rubble.

We, along with every ER in the city, kept waiting for more victims, but they just didn't materialize. Right away we started hearing about all these people that we knew in the NYC Fire Department who were missing.

Over the next twenty-four hours we had word that there were other burn patients at St. Vincent's and NYU Downtown who were ready to be transferred to us. Three days later we had twenty critical ventilated burn patients. That's a huge number of critical burn patients. They were all one-to-one, which meant one nurse was assigned to each patient. Remember, the dressing changes alone take two-and-a-half hours each.

These patients were conscious when they came in, but we had a pharmacist who dispensed the morphine and Ativan like it was candy. The volume of these drugs that we went through that day was tremendous—out of sight.

We had to be very careful about keeping the TVs in the patient's rooms turned off. Most of these patients didn't know that the buildings had collapsed, and we didn't want to tell them because we didn't know the affect it would have on them.

Out of the eighteen burn victims we received, eight died. Two of our victims were actually on the eighty-sixth floor. One badly burned man who survived told us that his coworkers who helped him down the stairs kept telling him that he only had ten more floors to go when he really had seventy. He made it out and collapsed.

By the second day we had most of the burn victims. The dilemma was that we didn't have the number of burn nurses we needed to care for that many patients. The survivors were going to be with us for a long time and were going to need intense twenty-four hour care. Our staff alone wasn't going to be able to handle that volume, so it was a good thing for us that people came out of the woodwork to help.

FEMA got involved and sent us nurses from Massachusetts General burn unit, and a few from other burn units across the country. We had a total of fifty-three nurses come through the unit who would stay anywhere from ten days to two weeks. They received IDs and quick, down-and-dirty "here's-how" instructions.

I was working sixteen hours a day for weeks. I'd go home and I'd try not to turn on the TV, but I just had to. Then I'd bawl my eyes out for an hour, go to sleep and be back at work early the next morning.

My supply budget for September and October was the largest I've ever seen. In those two months, we made over fifty thousand IV drips. We lived in the hospital around the clock. The stamina of my staff and the outside nurses was amazing. In all my years of nursing I've never seen such dedication.

Still, I started feeling like there was never going to be an end to it. It wasn't until mid-October that I realized the chaos wasn't going to last forever. At the end of October we cut back and went back to our regular staff. By then, some of the victims had died and some had improved.

I'll never forget the first victim who left the hospital—he was young and got through his initial recovery in about three weeks. It was such a major media event that I don't think there was a reporter, or a TV or radio station that didn't show up to record the event.

There was an outpouring of generosity from restaurants and churches, so no nurse ever had to leave the hospital to eat. We had everything from bottled water to gourmet food. We received thousands of cards and letters from all over the world. They covered every corridor in the hospital ceiling to floor.

February 2002

I've been to the site three or four times and to this day I cannot believe those towers are gone. It's nothing but a big hole in the ground. I had a favorite place at Bleeker Street and Lafayette and you'd look south and the towers would just loom. Now when you go there, there's nothing but a big empty space.

I think it will happen again. There are terrorists all around us, and to be honest, I don't think our nation has done enough for our security.

I don't live thinking that I have a lot of years a head of me. By that I mean that I take nothing for granted. I wake up every morning and wonder what I'm going to hear when I turn on the radio. Will it be the Empire State Building? The UN?

I see a day as a day. I'm here today—I don't know about tomorrow. I'm a churched man and I've grown a lot in my faith. I thank God for every day I have on this planet, because truly we don't know what will happen today or tomorrow.

MARIAH

"In my family, I'm a fourth generation nurse. I've worked med-surge, ICU, heart transplant, and ER, and I can tell you flat out that ER nurses stand apart from the rest.

"In order to be an ER nurse, you have to be self-assured and very knowledgeable. If you don't have those things, you aren't going to be able to keep ahead of the pressure. You will eventually make a fatal mistake, be fired, or burn yourself out.

"ER is a different ballgame—upstairs in the units the patients are already patients. They're in a nice bed in a clean gown and they have the patient mindset.

"In the ER, these people come in bloody or sick yet they don't accept themselves as patients. They just want to get treated and go home, even if they're critical and about to die. ER nurses have the task of getting them to accept the transition from being a person in control of their own destinies to a patient with a definite diagnosis.

"How are we supposed to unwind from the horrors we deal with all day? I'll come home around 1 a.m. and suddenly realize, 'Oh my God, I haven't peed today', or, 'Oops! I haven't eaten for sixteen hours.' It's no wonder why some nurses become closet drug addicts.

"I used to debrief with my husband, but he's not a medical person. All that stuff grosses him out. I mean, how do you describe

to a non-medical person about that patient who had a twelve inch butcher knife sticking out of his chest and not have them say, 'Oh euew! Stop.' "

One night we had a guy walk in off the street after stabbing himself through the chest with a twelve-inch carving knife. He was talking, lucid and calm—well, okay, maybe he was a little pissed off because he'd failed at what he was trying to do, but still he was pretty normal, considering.

The blade had nicked one of his ventricles so we were tiptoeing around this knife, treating it like a bomb ready to go off. I was trying to get a large-bore IV catheter into him before he went to surgery, but it was close to impossible because his blood pressure was dropping lower by the minute.

While I probed for anything resembling a vein, he casually talked to me about his garden. As we talked about what fertilizer he used on his roses, the wooden handle pulsated with every beat of his heart. It was mesmerizing. For weeks afterward, I had nightmares about that pulsating knife handle, to the point where I'd wake up in a sweat and have to walk around the house until the terror of it passed.

ER nurses are supposed to be tough. They aren't supposed to take on any of the emotional violence that we deal with every day. That's bullshit. For each trauma I get during a shift, I am also traumatized.

My nightmares come from things like the night they brought in a four-year-old whose mother had dragged him to the middle of a bridge and threw him off. She waited until he hit the water then jumped too.

The child was dead when they retrieved him from the water, so in reality, he should have been treated like a regular jumper who was dead at the scene. He should have gone to the morgue. But, because he was just a child, the paramedics felt they had to do *something*.

With a trauma like that, a medical professional's rationalization skills go out the window. Medical people automatically think, *He's only a baby. He has to survive. I have to do the best I can.* In the case of the paramedics, it's a matter of, "I'll do what I can and then hand him off to others who will save him."

Contrary to popular belief, people who jump off high places don't lose consciousness on their way down. They don't die until they hit the water or the pavement. That child had to have been terrified. Why the hell couldn't she have held him and jumped, just to have given him that last bit of comfort before death?

The cops told us the witnesses said the child had been screaming, "Please mommy, no! I promise I'll be good." when she threw him off. To this very day, whenever an abused child comes in, those words reverberate around my head.

In my whole career I have refused only once to take care of a patient. He was a nationally famous serial killer who came in from prison with chest pain. I knew immediately he was faking it and refused to be manipulated.

Because of what I see in the ER, I admit I have a touch of the eye for an eye mentality. All I could think was, *Here's the killer of fifteen innocent young women and he has more rights in my emergency room than any of those girls did at the time he was sadistically torturing them to death. And this inhuman monster is demanding* my *energy and attention?*

He gets free drugs, hot meals, and all the free dental and medical care he demands. What did those women and their families get?

Out of respect for his victims, I would not take part in supplying him with the pleasure of a nice drug high every time he got bored with prison.

Manipulators are the pits. They're the people who come in for drugs or a nice place to sleep. We have drunks and druggies coming in all the time. We give them IV nourishment and clean them up because they've puked, shit and peed all over themselves or have maggots crawling around their wounds.

We literally hand them the resources—find them jobs, places to live, give them medical and psychological help—you name it. At the time they're grateful, but two days later they're back just as screwed up and filthy and down and out as before. I give first and second chances to these people, but after that, forget it. I'm done.

I've been physically assaulted a few times during my years in the ER. I've bitched and moaned forever about nurse safety and even petitioned for a lockdown policy so the ER staff can seal themselves off from the rest of the building if a crazy wanders in with weapons and decides to blow a few nurses and doctors away. However, never in my wildest dreams did I imagine that my biggest threat would be a physician.

Somewhere along the course of my career I made a decision that I would never allow anyone—not a friend, or my husband, or a bum on the street—to talk to me in the same way physicians speak to nurses.

In my hospital, the physicians have been pampered and catered to for so long, they think they can get away with anything.

On a day that we were overwhelmingly busy, Dr. Q, the neurosurgeon on call for the ER that day, came in to consult on a patient who had had a significant head vs. baseball bat collision.

As I walked into the main room, I heard Dr. Q verbally abusing our clerk about a chart that he felt was not assembled correctly.

After he'd yelled for the third time that she was a "goddamned stupid pissant," I intervened and quietly asked him to please lower his voice because the patients were beginning to notice and get upset. Immediately, he turned his rage on me, shouting that I was a "meddling incompetent bitch."

That didn't bother me as much as the fact that the patients on the gurneys and treatment rooms closest to the ruckus were all watching this ER version of the Jerry Springer Show.

The rest of the staff stopped what they were doing and came to see what was going on.

In a pacifying gesture, I put up my hands and said, "Dr. Q, please calm down. We'll take care of your needs as soon as we can."

I didn't see it coming, and even if I had, I doubt I could have moved fast enough to avoid it. In a split second, Dr. Q had grabbed my arm and twisted it behind my back so that I fell to my knees. When he grabbed my throat, I snapped out of it and screamed for help. It took one nurse and two male patients to pull him off me.

I was still on the floor writhing in pain when the head nurse came to see what had happened. Standing over me she told me to be quiet and warned that I was not to tell anyone about the incident.

By the time I was sent to x-ray, I'd been presented with a written gag order by the director of nurses. The last thing the nurse-management liaison said to me as I was leaving to go home was, "Why all the fuss? It isn't as if the guy cut up your face or raped you. You came out of it with a small rotator cuff tear and some hurt pride—big deal. Get over it."

Despite fourteen written statements from witnesses, all corroborating what happened, hospital management chose to support the doctor and go after me, charging me with provoking a physician and causing an unpleasant situation to get out of hand.

The hospital charged me with being a danger to patients and demanded I see a psychiatrist they hired.

In an unexpected and happy twist of events, the psychiatrist at that evaluation advised me to call the police and charge the doc with assault and battery. I took his advice and the physician was convicted. The hospital was required to fine the doctor two hundred dollars, but they never did.

I, however, was put on probation, demoted, took a cut in salary, and threatened with losing my job if I took the matter any further. My whole career turned around that day. My goal of wanting to make my ER the best trauma center in the state changed to total apathy.

Now, I go in, I do my best for the patients and I go home. For me that's all there is that matters anymore.

DANIEL

"I left engineering when I was twenty-one and went into nursing with the help of my twin brother, who is a nurse clinical specialist.

"Growing up, I'd had good male role models who were nurses, so I never thought of it as a gay man's profession. Of course, there were issues within my family, my dad being a macho Latino, but my brother and I didn't give them any leeway, we just drove forward.

"I love the science of nursing and the whole idea of working on the frontlines to see how theory met actuality.

"I started looking seriously at becoming a doctor a year out of nursing school. I saw early on how the nurses and doctors interacted, and I thought there had to be a more cohesive way to go about that. I had a picture in my mind of how everyone could have fun and the patient could benefit.

"When I did become a doc, I didn't lose the compassion I'd found as a nurse. Because of that, I was constantly catching shit from the other docs because the patients would come in asking for me and refusing to see any of them.

"I doubt those doctors really care what it is I do that makes the patients react that way to me and not them, but then again, they're doctors, so they act in a manner they believe all doctors should—arrogant and above it all.

"My ideal view of the medical world would be to have doctors be nurses first. The hospital bean counters have been telling nurses for years that they could train baboons to do their job. Now the bean counters say the same thing about doctors. And to be honest, with some of the doctors I've seen, I'd have to agree.

"Me? Well, there's a big part of me that still thinks I'm a nurse so I don't really care what the hell the doctors think. I can't save them. These are not the type of people I want to go out drinking with after work. When I see other docs abusing a nurse out of their own arrogance, I always make sure I rip them a new asshole.

"Basically, the difference between being a nurse and a doctor for me is that as a nurse, you can see others making clinical decisions and you can follow along or not. As the doctor you have to generate the decision. If you're lucky enough to have nursing colleagues who can help you make those decisions, you're set. My favorite saying in residency was, 'You can kill some of the people some of the time, but try not to kill all the people all the time. Trust the nurses and you won't kill anybody any of the time.'

"If I were going to go back into nursing, I'd choose ER nursing again. I love the intervention and the immediacy of it. I love the stop and go of it. I love the fact that the ER is the patient's best chance of survival. I learned a lot about that when I served in Kuwait—patch up the holes first, and then run in the blood as fast as you can. Everything else is secondary."

The kid was 19. He came to our small ER from the construction site where he'd been working. He kept saying, "I fucked up, man, I really fucked up. It's all my fault. I talked the operator into letting me ride across the ditch on the rake of the backhoe."

Still, it didn't look like too much damage had been done, which was in line with what I'd been told had happened. According to the foreman, the boy had climbed onto the rake of the backhoe, and as the arm of the backhoe came across, it hit the wall of the ditch, pinning the boy across his mid-section just under his ribs. The dirt gave way immediately, so it was no big deal, right?

We didn't have the support of a big hospital, though the ER doc who was on at the time was one hell of a sharp internist. She knew enough to get a bunch of lines into him, and she kept looking at the kid with this really worried expression. Every few minutes she'd turn to me and say, "We need a surgeon, Dan. We need a surgeon in here now."

That didn't make sense to me at the time, because the kid was talking to us non-stop. He was lucid and he looked so good. I didn't have enough ER expertise under my belt yet to understand about sensitive bellies.

I kept my eye on the monitor and pretty soon I noticed that his heart rate was speeding up. But, he was still talking and lucid. I kept thinking, *What the hell is the problem here?*

Following instinct, I rolled him onto his side to do a back assessment and there was a trickle of blood leaking from his rectum.

The internist looked at me with a pained expression and whispered, "There's the problem."

The surgeon on call was in the middle of a case at the hospital across town, and the surgeon who was not on call, was out riding horses, so they sent someone to find him and bring him in.

What has always stuck with me was the way this kid's life just ebbed away. Right in front of us he grew weaker by the minute, getting more and more tired. He had no clue that he was dying.

Finally he said, "I'm tired. I'm going to go to sleep now," closed his eyes, and lost his pressure.

I started CPR in disbelief that this strong, muscular guy was going down. I jumped on the gurney and went with them into the OR, doing CPR the whole way. The surgeon opened his chest, took a feel around, then took my hand and wrapped it around the kid's flat heart with nothing in it. There was a big hole all the way through the aorta. I could actually stick my finger through the hole.

Thirty minutes into it, they let him go.

It was the first time I'd ever dealt with anything like that—the first time I really realized how quick we could all go. I just thought he had a tummy ache and we could fix it.

I went home and sat staring at the wall, trying to figure out what we could have done. I could not get over that he'd been so alive, and then he was dead. That perfect young life gone in a split second. I thought about all the things medical warriors think about when we've lost someone—if only the surgeon could have gotten there sooner, or if only we'd seen the blood right away, or if only he'd had his leg crushed instead. It just about did me in.

My rescue from the dark depression that enveloped me came a few weeks later in the form of my twin brother. He'd been through similar situations and he really helped me come to terms with that young man's death.

My brother decided that I needed some levity in my life. We'd always been brutal with each other about pulling practical jokes, and he knew my work schedule, so he thought it would be great fun if he sent me a dozen red roses a full shift ahead of when I was scheduled to work.

When I came in that day, one of the other nurses walked up to me, her eyes like saucers and said, "Ah, Dan, I think you should go to the staff lounge and check out the roses you received this morning."

In the lounge I found twelve long-stemmed roses sitting right out for everyone to see. Attached was a postcard-sized note that read:

Daniel Darling,

Last night bouncing around on the bed with you all in leather was fantastic! We'll have to do that again soon!

Next time, don't forget the feathers.

Love, Lance

I spent the rest of the shift trying to convince the other nurses that it was really just my twin brother playing a terrible practical joke, but they didn't believe me.

So, everybody in this small midwestern town—and you know what progressive souls midwesterners were in 1987—thought I had a gay lover in leathers. What really cemented that idea in everyone's mind was the fact that I'd made it a rule never to date any of the women who worked at the hospital.

However, I did get even with my brother. In our ER files, I found a psych consult report on a patient who'd been diagnosed as having deviant psychotic behavior. On the top of the report was a warning to restrain as necessary.

I obliterated the patient's name, substituted my brother's name and faxed it to the nursing station on his unit.

JAY CIVELLO
St. Vincent's Hospital, ER nurse
New York City resident

"I knew from the time I was a kid that I wanted to do something in healthcare. I started as a hospital volunteer at fourteen. At fifteen, I took a nursing assistant program. At sixteen, I became a nursing assistant.

"I thought what nurses did was more interesting than what the doctors did. The doctors seemed too mechanical, not really involved with the patients. The nurses got to know the patients.

"From the beginning, I wanted to work in the ER. Even though I love the uncontrolled atmosphere of an emergency room, I have some old fashioned values from the Catholic Hospital where I trained. I'm a very spiritual person and I bring this into my practice. It gives me the support I need to deliver the level of care that I want to give.

"September 11 was weird because it was all happening right in front of me. You want surreal? Surreal is triaging patients outside in the street, looking at the World Trade Center towers in flames, then taking a patient back for treatment and returning less than twenty seconds later, and seeing nothing except a plume of smoke where the tower used to be. Let me tell you, that *is* surreal.

"But you know, I never panicked. I've been an ER nurse too long to panic. One thing ER nurses never forget: we get paid to act, not react."

September 11, 2001
Manhattan, New York City

It was my day off. I'd worked nightshift the night before, so I was sound asleep when my sister called to tell me a plane had just hit the World Trade Center. I turned on the TV, saw the one tower on fire and immediately called the hospital. The clerk picked up the phone, heard my voice and said, "Get here! Get here now!"

It took me exactly four minutes to get out of bed, throw on sweat pants, grab my scrubs and get out the door and onto my bike. As I was peddling, I was thinking that it was only a small plane, but as I turned onto Fifth Avenue, I could see both buildings were ablaze.

On the corner was a group of Spanish newsboys on their knees making the sign of the cross and crying. That was when I realized that something catastrophic had happened.

As soon as I walked into the ER, people told me that the city was under attack. After checking in with our director and nurse manager, I was given the title of triage officer.

No one could get through to the ER without first going through triage first. We were to tag everyone, even if they were dead. It was such a strange concept to do it that way—no hands-on, no assessments, no nothing. I'd just ask the patient or EMT what the problem was, tag them, place them on a gurney or in a wheelchair, and then designate an area in the ER where they were to be taken.

It got crazy in that first hour or two. The patients were coming in six or seven to an ambulance. We saw eye irritations, smoke inhalations, burns, major trauma, people having chest pain from running down eighty flights of stairs, and people who made it out of the building, but had fallen running.

At some point we were given disaster bulletins that said the staff would have to remain on duty until further notice and would not be permitted to leave the hospital. Then we were given another notice from the Medical Examiner's office. I'll read it to you:

Policy regarding disaster fatalities: Any body received DOA should immediately be placed into a body bag and not be touched examined or photographed. The bag should then be marked with a permanent marker: 'D' for disaster, 'M' for Manhattan.'

The city had set up an area where the bodies would go even before the buildings fell, but there weren't a lot of bodies removed that first day.

I remember when the first building collapsed, there was an unreal hush throughout the ER. Everyone in the department was quiet and straight-faced. I was numb. Don't forget, everything was happening right down the block from us. I saw a one-hundred-and-ten-story building fall in Manhattan with my own eyes. I knew that no one was going to survive that. I mean, where do one hundred and ten stories *go*?

For a week afterwards, the hospital was on disaster mode—everyone thought that pockets of survivors would be rescued. For myself, I went off disaster mode the moment those buildings fell.

In the midst of all this, Mayor Giuliani came in saying that there was an estimated forty thousand people in those buildings, and I remember thinking, *Oh my God, how will we possibly do this?*

When we heard the Pentagon had been hit, I automatically figured we were at war and were going to be bombed again. I went into the triage booth and tried to call my family. Considering where I live and work, I knew they'd be worried. The phones, including my cell phone, were all dead. My family would have no way of knowing if I was alive or dead and my fear was that my mother might have a heart attack.

Then all the traffic stopped. It was like a strange nightmare. The fact we didn't get lots of patients bothered me for another reason other than it meant the loss of thousands of lives. To be honest, I was disappointed.

What I mean by that is, for those eighteen years of working in an ER, I'd lived for the moment of having a real disaster. ER nurses are like soldiers who train for combat—we're trained for disasters. I was ready to fight that day. Out of the three hundred sixty-five days a year that we put up with all that other junk like sore throats and ear aches, that day was our day to make a difference. All of us wanted to be so busy that our heads would spin—but it didn't happen.

Yes, we saw a lot of victims, but the majority of victims who we would have seen had the buildings not collapsed, didn't make it. *Those* were the people we could have helped.

About 5 p.m. we rotated taking breaks. Two other nurses and I took a walk in the opposite direction of the World Trade Center, into the little side streets. We walked and cried, knowing we'd lost people we knew and worked with every day.

I tried to make the other two nurses laugh by saying, "Look at it this way, we got to kick out the regulars. We got to throw them right out of the ER. Can you imagine? A dream come true! The usual down-and-outers were all there, and we got to say to them for the first time ever, "Hey you! Get outta' here! You can't come into my ER and abuse me today."

I finally got through to my mom's house. My sister answered and told me that everyone was there, asking if I was okay. I told her I was fine, but numb.

Then she said, "Jay, we're very proud of you, and we all just want you to know that."

I burst out crying. I couldn't tell you why. I never cry at my job, except once when somebody lost their child and I broke down with them. The next time I cried was a week after September 11 when I went to my mother's house. As soon as she saw me, she started hysterically crying, which set me off crying again.

September 12, 2001
1:30 a.m.

I went home, slept for a few hours, showered and went back to the ER. We saw mostly rescue workers although we did see some of the few survivors who'd been in the buildings.

In trauma and disaster situations, it's a natural instinct to run for home, which is what a lot of the people who managed to get away from the buildings did. Some of the commuters ran as far as the Brooklyn Bridge to get home.

There are two images I will never forget. One was the fireman who came in after the buildings collapsed, completely covered in that white dust. He fell to his knees and begged, "Please, please just wash my eyes out and let me go back down there. I have to get my coworkers out."

I understood that just waiting around to be seen would be pure torture for him, so I irrigated his eyes and let him go.

The other image that sticks with me was of this one woman who came in that night in complete traumatic shock, totally oblivious to where she was. She kept seeing the buildings falling on her. She had been in one of the towers and managed to get out, but as she turned around to look at the building, it started to fall. She ran, looking over her shoulder.

That's how she came in—lying on the stretcher with her head turned, looking behind her and screaming, "It's falling! Run! It's falling!"

She did that for hours. She'd look right at people, but not see them—she was looking through them. Then she'd try to run and hold onto something. It was horrible. They had to give her huge amounts of sedation to get her out of it.

That first night, the families sat on the curbs all the way down the block for as far as you could see. They were three and four people deep, holding candles and pictures of their loved ones.

If the nurses or doctors walked outside the hospital, they'd come up to us begging, "Have you seen this person?"

We didn't have any John or Jane Does, so all I could do was give them emotional support. It was very trying. It got so that I didn't want to leave the hospital for those first couple of days because I knew that the second I crossed that barricade, they'd be on me, begging, and I had nothing to give them.

My way of dealing with them was to look at the photo or the name and say, "No, that person doesn't look familiar to me." I'd then suggest that they might pray about it.

On the side of our hospital is a wall that's dedicated to the photos of these people. We call it the Wall of Hope and Remembrance. We still light the candles around it every day.

February 2002

I've opted not to go to Ground Zero. I love New York. It's my home. I'm a city boy—don't put me in a cabin on a lake—I'd never get to sleep with all that peace and quiet going on. I'm active in my community and I love New Yorkers—they're a unique breed of people. They're tolerant and non-judgmental.

To me, going down to Ground Zero would be like acknowledging defeat. I'm not going to look at it until it's rebuilt.

To be honest, I don't know if September 11 has changed my life forever. See, I have this joke that I always tell, that if I had my choice of coming back as anyone, I'd come back as me.

Sure, when I'm in the subway, I think twice about it, or if I hear a plane overhead, I do look up.

As far as the value of life, September 11 probably showed a lot of people that life is precious and they need to live every moment. Being an ER nurse, I've always known that life is short. We see little versions of September 11 every day. We know for a fact that no one can guarantee you will be here tomorrow or even in five minutes from now.

Being an ER nurse has showed me all along that life is precious. It goes with my philosophy that when I talk to my depressed friends, I say, "What do you mean you can't laugh and have a good time? I work in an emergency room and I can still laugh and have a good time."

I think about September 11 a lot. I can't imagine what it must have been like for those people, especially the ones who jumped to their deaths. I can barely look at those photos of the people hanging onto the windows before they jumped to their deaths. That conflict is not even conceivable to me. No living creature on this earth should ever be made to make a decision like that. I've had nightmares about those people jumping. They were all someone's loved one.

The support we got was tremendous. We received cards and gifts from ER staffs all across the country saying they were behind us. And all the patients who came in after that were full of appreciation.

But hey, lest I flower this up too much, let me also say that within a month, the patients were back to their old ways, saying the usual, "Hey, you! Shithead! Get over here and take care of me!"

I swear, sometimes I think we should get combat pay for what we do.

MICK

"I started out as a fireman working airport crashes, became an EMT, then a paramedic, and finally, an ER tech on the south side of Chicago. I married one of the ER nurses and decided to go to nursing school.

"As far as I was concerned, nursing school was worthless. They stressed the most ridiculous things, like two weeks on how to make a bed instead of teaching the really useful bedside skills like what to do when your patient stops breathing.

"I've been a nurse for eight years and in all that time I have never had any gender issues with anybody, although I have noticed the physicians are more polite to me than they are to the female nurses. They'll belittle a female nurse but would never try that on me, and it has nothing to do with the fact I'm six-feet-four and weigh over three hundred pounds.

"Female nurses simply don't stick together when it comes to forcing a positive change. A few years ago the nurses in my hospital were given the opportunity to vote for a union. They voted it down, and the hospital gave them free pizza. Believe me when I tell you men would never have voted it down even for a free, solid gold pizza.

"If I had to pick one thing that I've learned from ER nursing, it would be that I try not to let anything negative stay with me. If my wife and I have a fight, I'm always quick to fix it, because she or I *could be dead in the next minute. People just don't realize how fragile life really is."*

It was my first week in ER. I was a new grad, so they didn't want to give me any patients who were too challenging, thus limiting the chance of my killing or hurting anybody. Most of the patients assigned to me had simple, straightforward diagnoses like sprains, lacerations, flu or pneumonia. So when this seventy-year-old lady with a bad case of bronchitis and flu came in, she was all mine.

I did my initial assessment and took her for a chest x-ray. She was pretty dehydrated from not being able to hold any liquids down, so the doc ordered that a hydrating IV with some antibiotics be run in right away.

While I was starting the intravenous line, we chatted about her grandkids and her garden and how she loved to play bingo at her church. As I recall, she was really into the whole bingo thing, because she got so excited about it, I had to steer her to some other subject. She did tell me however, that she played six or seven Bingo cards at a time, so I figured she had to be pretty sharp.

By most social standards, she was lucid, alert, and quite normal, which is more than I can say for ninety percent of the patients we see.

I moved on to my next patient, and about a half-hour later I returned to the old lady's treatment room to check on her IV. It was hard not to notice that she was agitated and muttering obscenities under her breath. There was no trace of her previously sweet and cheerful demeanor. In just thirty minutes, she'd changed from an endearing, bingo-playing church lady to Cruella de Vil.

Thinking she might be having an adverse reaction to the antibiotic, I slowed her IV and did another set of vital signs. When I saw that everything was within normal range, I chalked her agitation up to the hospital atmosphere, and passed it off.

I charted her vital signs and as I was leaving the room, she yelled at the top of her lungs, "And keep those goddamned clowns out of my room! I hate clowns! Tell them to do their fucking cartwheels in somebody else's room!"

My first thought was, "Okayyyyy, I guess I better report that her orientation level has slipped a few notches." I had the clerk page her doctor, then told the charge nurse that the lady was getting confused and we probably needed to get a blood oxygen level to make sure she was getting enough oxygen to her brain. I checked through her history to make sure we hadn't overlooked something, but there was nothing about her being confused or having any issues with dementia previous to this ER visit.

When her physician returned my call, I explained that his patient had hallucinated seeing clowns in her room. He was totally baffled. The woman, a longtime patient of his, had never before exhibited any signs of dementia, and none of the medications we'd given her could have caused the confusion. He ordered some stat blood work and said he'd be right in to check on her.

As I turned to tell the clerk what the doc had ordered, five clowns in full clown regalia came cartwheeling through the center of the ER lobby.

That day we submitted a formal request to administration to please warn us the next time they recruited volunteers from the local clown school to cheer up the patients.

ANONYMOUS
Ground Zero

"The only reason I work as an ER nurse is because it's a diversion. I think ER nursing is a thankless job. I respect the nurses who work ER, but I have to be honest, my first loyalty goes to working in the field as a paramedic.

"As a paramedic I do a lot of things nurses aren't allowed to do. In New York City, the action is not in the emergency rooms, it's on the streets. I did my time in the South Bronx and Harlem, so I know this first hand. If I'd been working in ER as a nurse on 9/11, the only thing I would have been doing was waiting for patients who never arrived.

"The saddest photograph I saw of 9/11 was of all these medical professionals lined up outside St. Vincent's, waiting to help. I specifically remember the photo of a doctor sitting on the curb holding a laryngoscope, with his head in his hands. It was like they were all there for nothing. Not that they didn't treat some patients, but it must have been a tremendous frustration.

"For the last few months, I've been working on finding photos or videos of the people who were working down at the World Trade Towers during those last few minutes. If we can find one picture of a husband, father or brother who was working to save others, it will give much better closure to the family than having nothing.

"As a paramedic, I was bombarded by the press initially—they were rabid about getting our stories about what was going on down at the site. It was hard not to notice that the nurses—as usual—were completely overlooked."

September 11, 2001
New York City
Ground Zero

I'd planned on sleeping in, but I couldn't sleep. I got up, poured myself a cup of coffee and turned on the TV at the same moment a reporter broke in to say that a twin-engine plane had crashed into the World Trade Center. I remembered the World Trade Center bombing incident back in 1993, and thinking it couldn't be too bad, called my unit to make sure that was the case.

As soon as my supervisor answered, he started yelling that I needed to come in right away. When I arrived at Broadway and Fulton, people were attempting to stage the ambulances by lining them up for transporting victims. Because of the amount of debris that was falling, and the extreme nature of the fire, I made the decision to pull everyone back even though it wasn't what we'd normally do in the case of multiple casualty incidents.

In New York City, the way we are taught to fight high-rise fires is to treat the patients on the floor below the fire, so if the fire is on the tenth floor, you'll be on the ninth floor treating the victims. At the very least, we should have been triaging the patients in the lobbies of the towers, but I decided to set up our triage across the street just outside the Millennium Hotel. We only had our turnout gear, not bunker gear, so our stuff wasn't fireproof.

We classified the patients in terms of injury: the walking wounded were green tagged, the less serious with yellow, the most critically injured with red, and the dead with black. So as not to waste our resources, our goal was to save who could be saved, and leave the most critically injured behind.

I was appointed to make sure that the seriously injured people were transported. At the time, we were taking only the badly burned patients in our ambulances. We couldn't take all the patients because there were so many. I remember looking up at the buildings and thinking that we probably hadn't even begun to see the most serious patients because the firefighters hadn't had time to get them down to us.

That was when I saw this one woman lying in the middle of the street. Normally officers aren't supposed to get involved in patient care, but I wanted to get her out of the street, so I called over a couple of EMTs to help.

We were carrying her out of there when I heard a high-pitched screeching noise that had an underlying thunder to it. Some people thought it was a nuclear blast, but I thought it was a low flying plane coming in to destroy the remaining survivors. Even though anything was possible at that point, nobody thought it was the sound of the World Trade Center collapsing.

One of the EMTs screamed at us to run. There was no time to take any patients, so we dropped the woman we were carrying and started running. We left a lot of patients at that triage site. I don't know how many of them died. I can't think about that.

When I got to Fulton Street, I looked over my shoulder in time to see a mountainous cloud of debris coming right at me. I was overtaken by it just as I made it to Broadway. I reached for the wrought iron fence surrounding St. Paul's Chapel and prepared for the impact of the implosion concussion.

The second my hand grabbed the fence, a powerful wind hit me. I don't know how I was able to hold on, but I did. The strange thing was that after that horrendous blast of wind, there was complete and utter silence. Never in all my life could I remember the world being so silent. There was no question in my mind that I was going to die. It wasn't like a car accident where it's over in an instant—this was a drawn out, prolonged expanse of time in which you know you are going to be dead in a few moments.

I didn't want to die alone, so I reached out and said to someone next to me, "Please hold my hand." A woman took hold of my hand, and all around me I could hear voices saying very quietly, "I can't breathe. Please help me, I'm dying."

I tried to take a breath and couldn't because the air was solid with particles. It was pitch black and I knew in that instant that death was there for me, so I prayed to God to let me live. Just as I finished this small prayer, I saw a very bright light. I was wearing a helmet with a visor that partially covered my face, so I pulled my shirt up over the bottom of my face and began to breathe through the fabric. When I opened my eyes, the light was gone, and it was dark, but not as black as it had been, so I left there and started walking as fast as I dared.

It wasn't long before I found a small van with two men inside, both of whom were in bad shape and needed to get to a hospital. I got in and drove without being able to see much, but eventually, there was enough light for me to see where I was. Somehow I made my way to the hospital. Like the other two men in the car, I was having serious problems breathing.

In the ER one of the nurses started an intravenous line on me, and all I could think about was that I needed to go back down to the site to help. As soon as I could clear my airway and get my eyes irrigated, I ripped out my IV and went right back down to Ground Zero.

For the next twenty hours, I worked in the chaos of the rubble. Body parts were strewn everywhere. It felt strange working down there because I could feel the presence of those souls all around me. It was crazy down there. People stomped around without direction, cranes were moving constantly, and bulldozers were charging everywhere. I thought, *My God, we'll lose more rescue workers than victims in this insanity.*

I saw gruesome things at Ground Zero what with the jumpers and the body parts, but you know, I've seen worse. I've worked in some of the toughest neighborhoods in New York. It was nothing to see five shootings a night for weeks on end, or twenty cardiac arrests a week during heat waves. I've had little kids handed to me who had been stabbed, shot, choked and beaten to death by their own parents.

I've seen so many horrific things working in the city, that graphically, September 11 was not the worst thing I've ever seen. It was the enormity of the whole situation that was overwhelming. What I did and saw that day was just part of the job. I didn't think about it much at the time. It's like driving a car. You don't have to think about it, you just do it. I won't tell you it didn't affect me, but I will say I was very non-emotional about it while it was happening.

I couldn't tell you that now. A few days after it happened was probably the most emotional experience of my life. There has never been anything in my life that has fucked me up as much, or had such an enormous impact on me as the moment I fully realized the gravity of what had happened. I'd been working on the pile for about twenty hours, when I stopped to drink some water. I looked down, and saw a whole left arm with the hand still attached. There was a gold band on the ring finger. In a glance I knew everything about that person that I needed to know—that person had loved and been loved in return. And now, that person was gone forever.

I've seen the before and after collapse footage of those people working down there. I can tell you that if you really look at them and listen carefully, you'll see that people in disaster situations are very quiet. They aren't chatty. With the exception of the sound of the machinery, there's no noise. People weren't conversing with others—they were just doing what they had to do. They don't cry, they don't express emotion. They are zombie-like.

We worked twelve-hour shifts seven days a week for five weeks. You know what that does to you physically and psychologically? People were pretty depressed and burnt out and nobody was really eager to tell their story.

I haven't debriefed. I refuse to see a goddamned shrink because most shrinks are such voyeurs about all this shit. I say to them, "Go watch the TV if you want the ugly details. Don't charge me a hundred seventy-five bucks an hour to satisfy your morbid curiosity." The people who were there don't want to talk about this with anyone anymore.

Yes, I have loyalty to my country, but I never felt anger, not for one second. I couldn't go there. I am just thankful to be alive. The one thing that was reinforced in me that day was that we are in control of nothing. If you really believe you are in control, you're in need of some serious therapy. As individuals and as a nation we were in control of nothing, because no matter how great of a nation we were, or how strong we were as people, we were being controlled by something else that day.

Do I believe in God? Absolutely. God saved my life. I didn't live through that day because of anything else. Believe me—it is true that there are no atheists in the foxhole.

SUE AVERILL
ER nurse, Ebola Treatment Center
Freetown, Sierra Leone, Africa

"When I was a little kid, for as far back as I can remember, I knew I wanted to be a nurse. I don't know where that came from; there were no nurses in my family, I didn't know anyone who was a nurse, and at that age I hadn't read or seen anything about nurses—I'm not even sure I knew what a nurse was. Still, there was never any doubt in my mind that I would be a nurse. It was always part of who I was and who I wanted to be.

"In nursing school, for my final semester practicum I decided to work in ER so I could see everything. It didn't take long before I knew ER was in my blood. I got loads of experience in those three and a half months. Because of a major walkout by the ER nurses, I was hired two weeks before my graduation as charge nurse because I was the most experienced nurse there. I was twenty-three years old.

"ER nursing is challenging. It brings together one's knowledge, skills, intuition, diplomacy, compassion, and doggedness—all qualities good and bad. Once in motion we can adjust or change course, step over obstacles, bypass walls. We learn to make decisions and live by the results. We accept fear and anxiety as part of what gives us an edge. We see the worst of people and the best. Many times we are frustrated and vow to quit, but ER is in one's DNA—at least it has been in mine for thirty-five years.

"I've done a number of missions over the years with Doctors Without Borders, starting in Darfur in 2004, and I feel that the Ebola outbreak is probably the biggest health crisis we've had in our adult lifetimes. There are so few people available to go to these places and assist, that if I am in the position to be able to help, then it is my responsibility to get involved. The more I read and listened and learned, the less afraid I was of Ebola, and the more confident I was that I could work safely in the places that were affected and contribute to ending the outbreak.

"In 2007 I founded One Nurse At A Time, a non-profit organization that helps nurses become involved in volunteer work. We believe that nurses are the pebbles, which, when dropped into the pond, make far-reaching ripples. If we can put more nurses into the world, we will exponentially impact healthcare for those most in need."

EBOLA TREATMENT CENTER
FREETOWN, SIERRA LEONE, AFRICA

Wednesday, January 14, 2015
Day One

After a few days of training with Médecins Sans Frontières in Geneva, and a grueling journey to Sierra Leone, I enter the Ebola Treatment Center in Freetown where I will be working. At the entrance to the Ebola Treatment Center (ETC) compound, we get out of the car, wash our hands with 0.05% chlorine water, spray the bottoms of our shoes, and have our temperature taken. No one can enter the center until they go through this process.

Once allowed inside, we proceed to the entrance of the low risk zone—again, washing our hands and spraying our shoe bottoms. Then on to the dressing rooms—one side for men and one for women. In the dressing rooms we find our scrubs and hopefully, a pair of heavy plastic gumboots that fit. The scrubs and the boots will be washed and dried multiple times throughout the day.

From there we head over to the medical office tent where there is an area for administrative work and an area where we have hung white boards detailing each patient. There is another space set up for mixing IVs, etc., and another for the pharmacy folks who pack the med bags.

The ground inside the ETC is covered with jagged grey rock. Walking in my gumboots is uncomfortable and clumsy, but I'm sure I'll get used to that.

I spend the morning in triage, which I really like. However, the triage here is the reverse of American triage. Here, we don't respond to the sickest patients first, we respond first to those who are *not* sick, and get them out of the center with a certificate that says they do not have Ebola.

This is how it works: People come in and sit in a holding area consisting of plastic chairs two meters apart. This is considered the safe distance, which is the distance sputum can fly during a cough. The healthcare workers stand under a shade, behind an orange double fence blocking off two meters distance from them. There is no confidentiality as we call out to them, asking for their demographics and symptoms. It is here that we make a determination about whether or not to admit a person.

Today many had vague symptoms, but were relatives of confirmed Ebola patients—a husband, sister, and baby.

This is not unusual. We know the hot spots—those places where many of the positive cases are originating.

We admit a half dozen people. As we complete their paperwork, we give them a bag of water and a sachet of Plumpy'Nut, which is a highly nourishing peanut based paste loaded with calories, vitamins and mineral salts, and encourage them to eat and drink. Children like the Plumpy'Nut—the adults, not so much.

A psychologist comes and asks the patients if there is anyone they can call for them and if there is anything that needs to be done, such as finding a caretaker for their children. A Health Promoter talks to them about what's happening to them.

Oddly enough, the new patients are stoic. No comments, no questions. They just sit there across a far divide from us. The patients are then moved to another holding area and a nurse in full Personal Protective Equipment (PPE) comes to get them, take them to a bed, and get them settled.

The ambulances also come to the triage area. They back up halfway into the orange double fence area, then wait for the hygiene team to come spray the vehicle, remove the patient/stretcher, spray again, spray inside, then bring the patient to triage, where we do our work from across another two-meter table-like barrier. The only time we get any closer is with goggles or a face shield, when leaning close enough to take a temperature with the little electronic gun from six inches away.

There are separate areas inside the high-risk zone for suspected Ebola patients and confirmed Ebola patients. The patients who present with symptoms and/or fever, we admit to the suspect area. In the suspected area the patients are given a bed in a private room consisting of a concrete floor, walls of vinyl tarps, roof, sunshade, buckets for Oral Rehydration Solution (ORS), vomit, washing, and stool. We put the low suspect patients as far away from the high suspect patients as possible. The last thing we want is to expose someone who just has malaria to Ebola.

The suspect area is where the lab team, dressed in full PPE, draws blood for the Ebola blood test. The protocol just for drawing the blood is complicated. First the lab technician must write patient information on the blood tube, then they draw the sample, spray the outside of the tube, spray the inside of a zip lock bag, drop in the tube, spray the outside of the bag, spray the inside of another zip lock bag, drop in the tube and the first bag, then spray the outside of that second zip lock. All this goes into a solid blue container with chlorine solution inside and is hand carried about two blocks to the laboratory. Imagine doing all of that in the heat and humidity of this place.

The confirmed area also has a separate section for those with the highest nursing/medical needs. It is known as the ICU, the high-risk zone. It's not an ICU in the sense of what we have in America. Here, there are no machines, and no invasive care—just patients who need a close eye. These patients are so ill they cannot walk or drink by themselves. The children under five are especially vulnerable and have an 85 percent mortality rate. It is not easy seeing so many little ones die

Today I don full PPE and go into ICU to start IVs. Because I am good at starting IVs, I know I will be doing this more often.

There is also a third area for recovering convalescent patients. These people can walk, feed, and care for themselves. They have to test negative twice, plus be 72 hours without symptoms in order to be discharged home as cured. Caregivers for the children are recruited from these survivors because they seem to have immunity for an unknown period of time.

Things move slowly here. Since there is no such thing as an emergency, no resuscitation, no adrenaline-charged codes, we take our time to work out the best plan of action for everything.

Standard treatment is giving lots of fluids, antibiotics and anti-malarial drugs, correcting electrolyte imbalances, and supporting liver and kidney function. The end goal of any kind of treatment we give is to keep the patient alive for one more day, and then another and another while the body develops antibodies to fight the virus. It's really all about keeping the body alive, buying time for those antibodies to start working.

The ICU has a corridor down the middle with Plexiglas walls so we can literally walk down the middle without protective gear, and still be able to see and talk with our patients. This minimizes the time we spend in PPE. It's the same in the other wards, though not with Plexiglas. Instead, they have the two meter wide double fence, like in triage, so we can talk to the patients across it without having to be in PPE. There are also slanted one-way tables so we can pass them meds, food, or whatever they need. We slide it down to them across the two meters, or push it with a stick if necessary.

There are two slide tables at the entrance to the ICU as well, so that from the outside we can slide in another IV bag, tape, or whatever a nurse might need that they didn't take in with them.

Blood is drawn by the lab team three times a day. They process the samples in about four hours, so we can clear those who are not sick and send them out with their certificate.

Overall, I'm feeling pretty positive about this mission.

Friday, January 16, 2015
Day Three

My scrubs are saturated with sweat, although I have yet to experience pouring out half a boot of sweat like one of the doctors.

Today our numbers dropped. No new admissions, a few discharges cured! Happy dance.

There were several deaths. Our ratio since opening December 10 is about one cured to one dead. Mortality rate previously was up to 80 percent, so achieving 50 percent and under is really quite remarkable. Still, there is much more to be done.

I'm adjusting to the heat, drinking at least two gallons of water a day if not three. So far I'm scheduled for eight thirteen-hour shifts.

Hardest thing to manage right now is my feet. Those damned rubber boots are necessarily loose—so they provide no support, especially when worn for the full thirteen hours. The only time I don't wear them is when I go to lunch. My feet, knees and legs ache all the time despite Tylenol and ibuprofen.

The medical team is generally very nice. There are always people coming and going—Swiss, Mexican, German, Swedish, French, Italian and a couple of Americans.

This morning I must have washed my face a little too vigorously because I had a teensy nick on my chin, so I couldn't go into the high-risk zones. It will be healed tomorrow.

I'm happy to be here doing my best. Yesterday a sourpuss accused me of being an optimist. I laughed and said, "Yes I am!"

Tuesday, January 20, 2015
Day Seven

The good news: I got to sleep in until 9 a.m.! The bad news: I have to work a twelve-hour night shift for the first time in thirty-two years.

I've been working at the Ebola Treatment Center for a full week and I'm feeling pretty comfortable. During my training in Geneva I felt like a Frankenstein monster moving in the PPE suit, and now I'm relatively comfortable in it. Of course, comfort is a relative term. At this point in time I can safely dance a little jig in the suit and I'm getting used to drops of sweat running down my back, legs, neck, and face—especially from my upper lip into my mouth.

Our numbers are down. When I arrived a week ago, we had twenty patients in ICU and about fifty total. As of yesterday, we had nineteen total. Since December 10 there have been many deaths, but approximately forty-five to fifty survivors.

It's too early to know why the decrease. Are there really fewer cases? Is it because there are more beds available in more centers? Are people just not reporting in because their house will be quarantined by the military for twenty-one days and no one will be allowed to leave? Or, is the virus just taking a breath before it comes roaring back like it did last summer? The only time to safely let down our guard is once the twenty-one days have passed with no cases.

Right now we have seventeen-year-old M—, who is as wild as can be. One of the features of Ebola is incredible mental confusion and agitation, so despite Valium and Haldol, M— almost escaped from not only our ICU, but out of the triage area into the clean space as well. A couple of days ago, he nearly staggered into the decontamination shower.

Since we can only touch him in full PPE, the staff were shepherding him back to his bed with a long stick. If he should happen to rip the PPE suit, it poses a huge risk to the wearer.

Ebola survivors work for us in the high-risk areas, taking care of patients like M—. The survivor who took M— on for special attention, realized that he himself had been just as confused and threatening to the staff as M—. He's strong enough to manage M— and get him back into a chair or onto the mattress on the floor.

The confused patients are the hardest to manage. We work so hard to establish an intravenous line in them for the massive hydration they require, but as soon as you turn around, they pull out their IV and water and blood pour out everywhere. We can only be inside with the confirmed patients for one hour at a time, so it is quite discouraging.

I like staying busy and having to problem-solve. I like instilling the notion of critical thinking in the staff. Yesterday one of the nurses came up to say they were concerned because M— and one other young man have generalized edema and they wondered if too much IV fluid was being given. That's the first time they've come forward to question something like this, and I'm delighted.

My daily notes are always crumpled and soggy from sweat. By 7:30 a.m. the backs of my hands are forming droplets. When I take off the first layer of gloves in the PPE, I find there are several milliliters of sweat in each finger.

My feet are feeling a little better, but my legs and knees are still throbbing.

Saturday, January 24, 2015
Day Eleven

A man came to us with his brother, sister and new wife, whose mother had died of Ebola. Unfortunately, his wife was severely ill and died in a couple days despite our best efforts. The man and his sibling survived and today were discharged as cured.

The man was elated and spent half an hour with us saying thanks, wanting pictures taken. He tells us what he remembers during his illness: how hard it was to drink because he was so nauseated, how afraid he was in the night that he wouldn't live until morning, and how good he felt every time we went into his room to tell him he was doing well, and treat him kindly. He especially remembers me because of my blue eyes which are all that show through the PPE goggles.

Some of them are happy and dancing on their way out—until they find their homes empty, interior sprayed with chlorine and door locked, all possessions burned. No clothes, no mattress, no money to buy new things. Some of the community councils are doing this in an effort to stop the spread.

Everything the patients bring with them into the ETC is burned—cell phones (we can wash the SIM card in chlorine), belts, shoes, clothes. Logistics, the ETC support folks, buy clothes and shoes at the market so we can outfit the cured patients in a dignified way for going home.

Today we have two little ones in the suspected area. They are not doing well. One seized all night despite a lot of Valium IV. Both initially tested negative for Ebola, so they have to stay a couple of additional days to retest. It is probably malaria causing the high fevers, but we're struggling to keep them alive long enough to get that second test. We can transfer them to the pediatric hospital, but only when we confirm it is not Ebola.

A seventeen-year-old girl and an eight-year-old in ICU are not doing well. We move one darling five-year-old boy to the confirmed area. Poor dear is playing all by himself because the other children are too sick. He is now our resident doctor—he hung his toys on the IV hook and pretends he is giving himself a drip. So cute. Should have gotten a picture of that.

Celebrate the good and move past the sad.

Monday, January 26, 2015
Day Thirteen

It's been decided that the nurses can do the triage, screen patients in or out, write admitting orders, etc. I normally work ICU, but today and tomorrow I am in triage to cover the nurse who's working overnight shift.

I admit one man who looks sick, and indeed is positive with a high viral load. I also admit a child who is limp and reportedly had a convulsion last night. I am hoping he might be malaria instead, because he's had no contact exposure.

We end the day with a total of eighteen patients, which is probably a record low. Everyone is counting the outbreak over, but it's not yet, not until it's gone. Cases are not rising nor falling, more holding steady. I hear Liberia is doing much better.

Today there were lots of celebrations as three were discharged as cured, and five in the suspected area had negative blood tests.

Yesterday I had to pronounce a seven-year-old boy dead. It was especially sad because I'd been with him a couple hours before. Poor little guy.

Monday, February 2, 2015
Day Twenty

We went six days without a new confirmed case, but finally today we confirmed one—the ten-year-old brother of the man who was so grateful for himself and his siblings. I'm not sure why this family continues to be plagued. I assume the house has been decontaminated and they are well off and educated, so I am not sure why we continue to get infected siblings.

From triage, I admit nine new patients. I think two, possibly three, will be positive. No one looks especially sick, so hopefully they will all do well.

We have four confirmed cases total. That's down from a high of about fifty when I arrived. Overall, all three affected countries have reported very few new cases and it seems the outbreak emergency may be over. There might still be the odd case here and there. There is still a need for vigilance and surveillance and, of course, a place to appropriately treat the patients, but I think Médecins

Sans Frontières might be starting to fold up the tent and move on to the next crisis. There is always another crisis.

I hope some of the development charities come to help rebuild what's been devastated by this disease. I hope the reflection and review process finds lessons learned that can be applied to the next disaster. I hope the statistics and studies and research can lead to cures and early detection and better treatment modalities. I hope we can avoid another horrific loss of life as we've seen with this epidemic. I hope the world stops thinking, "If it's not my country/continent/people, I don't have to deal with it." I hope drug manufacturers and vaccine producers and the FDA all work together for people and not profit.

Wednesday, February 4, 2015
Day Twenty-two

Only three confirmed patients and two in suspect. Today the convalescent tent was torn down and burned. Only ten of the thirty suspect area beds are open.

It really seems the outbreak emergency is over. There is a thought that Ebola may now be endemic in the region with smaller outbreaks on occasion, or an isolated case here and there.

Earlier we had a period of six days with no new cases admitted, but then one by one they began to trickle in again. There were few deaths, which really helps morale.

Two of the expat nurses want to go home now. I was asked to stay, and said yes. In another week or so, there will only be three expat nurses and three expat doctors, so we won't be tripping over each other any longer!

A team has been formed to interview and do health exams for the survivors. The survivors say they love coming back to the ETC because we treat them like heroes (which they are) but in their communities they are still shunned. So far, one consistent thing is they all have shoulder pain. I am not sure why that is except that there is a lot of muscle damage from Ebola.

The president of Sierra Leone has promised to open schools again the second or third week of March. They have been closed since last July.

Friday, February 6, 2015
Day Twenty-four

I'm being sent home early along with two other nurses. Most of the doctors are also leaving in the next week, leaving two nurses and two doctors to do the closing down.

On Monday I will be debriefed, and on Tuesday, I fly westward to Seattle. Home. Then, I'll have twenty-one days of hanging out, taking my temp twice a day, but no isolation, no quarantine. I'm up for visitors, food, sleep, walks, and adult beverages.

I feel like I have personally and professionally accomplished what I set out to do. I think I contributed to the greater good of the Ebola effort and I helped advance the nursing practice among the Sierra Leonean staff. It's been hard work, but fun, too.

Afterword

For the last 35 years I have been repeatedly asked how nurses can bear to do what they do and why do they choose to deal with the horrors and the sorrows they see each day.

Since the why and how are essentially the same question, my stock answer to both has always been that nurses are able to do what they do because they are rich in the gifts of healing, compassion and love.

Several of the nurses in this book made statements to the effect of, "We are nurses—this is what we do; it is who we are." In that simple declaration is the better answer to the hows and whys.

Nursing is a calling. Not everyone can do it, and most people wouldn't want to, considering that it is one of the most difficult and demanding professions there is. Practicing the art of healing is not always well paid. It is physically and emotionally taxing, sometimes dangerous, and, it carries with it the responsibility of saving lives and easing suffering. The work is often stressful and at times, disheartening. In the course of a 12-hour shift, nurses deal with life-and-death events that, unless you live in a war zone, most non-medical people won't face but once or twice in a lifetime.

Most nurses are born to the profession, myself included. Signs of the emerging nurse can frequently be found in people while they are still very young. The individual who is drawn to nursing as a profession is often the child who nurtured pets, dragged home stray animals, and cared for sick and/or injured siblings or friends. For nurses whose family of origin was in some manner dysfunctional and stressful, they were the kids who were always trying to "fix" any injurious or uncomfortable situations in order to make things better.

Because these nurses grew up surrounded by chaos and drama-trauma, the mayhem and adrenaline rush that comes with working in the critical care arena, are, for them, a walk in the park.

I understand that this is dime-store psychology, but to explain the deeper whys and wherefores of those particular psychological dynamics is a whole other book.

Plainly put, nurses are *driven* to do what they do. For a nurse, caring and healing others is the most basic mode of being—it is their nature. This, when combined with education, skill, dedication, compassion and strength, makes nurses a powerful force. Recently I saw a T-shirt with the saying, "I'm a nurse. What's your superpower?" and had to laugh at the absolute truth of it.

Nursing is not for the weak or the faint-hearted. Of those who go lightly into nursing on a whim, or think of it as only a job and not a lifetime vocation, most will soon leave the profession or be drummed out one way or another.

Nurses have the power to touch and change people's lives in a profound way. Nurses save lives, ease suffering, and dispel anxiety and anguish. In return, they are rewarded with a deep sense of achievement, fulfillment and joy.

E.H.

Acknowledgments

I wish to thank the following nurses who shared their stories with the rest of us, and extend that gratitude to those others who provided help and support in making this book possible.

Peter Allar RN, Tracy Baughman RN, Patricia Bemis RN, Mary Jane Boyd RN, Amy Brown RN, Mary Carouba, Ann Carroll RN, Jay Civello RN, Bob Dembiki RN, Melissa Doherty RN, Lorraine Ensminger RN, Victoria Errico RN, Liz Froneberger RN, Rachael Garrity—book design expert, Judy Gavin RN, Carl Ginsburg—New York State Nurses Association, Michael Gross, Esq. of Author's Guild legal team—for his astute legal counsel, Kathleen Hollowed RN, Chuck Idelson—California Nurses Association, Rich Kavanagh RN, Frank Langben, Angel Lopez RN, Connie Baxter Marlow, Shirley Marshall RN, Kathleen McClure—copyeditor deluxe, Nancy Issing McGuire RN, Debbie McKellar RN, Suzanne Pugh RN, David Ramos RN, Rita Reynolds RN, Sereta Robinson, Colin A. Ross, Ann Schott, Steven M. Stowe, Laura Gasparis Vonfrolio RN, Mary Watters, Lucille Yip RN, Anonymous, and to Sue Averill, RN, who so generously gave me permission to use excerpts from her blog posts at www.OneNurseAtATime.org.

And last but not least, I wish to shower gratitude upon my one-in-a-million husband, Steven Vermillion, for his extraordinary patience, kindness, and especially for his ability to make me laugh.

About the Author

Echo Heron is the *New York Times* bestselling author of *Intensive Care: The Story of a Nurse* and eight other books, including *Tending Lives, Condition Critical, Mercy, Noon at Tiffany's,* and the Adele Monsarrat mystery series *Pulse, Panic, Paradox,* and *Fatal Diagnosis.*

Praise for Echo Heron

TENDING LIVES

"A convincing portrait of nursing as a beleaguered but honorable profession full of weary, caring men and women. Reveals in a sometimes shocking and sometimes comical fashion what the caring profession is really like. Enlightening . . . unsettling . . . compelling reading."
—*Kirkus Reviews*

"Deeply involving. The inside story of unforgettable medical dramas. (Heron's) sharp wit and indomitable spirit comes through again."
—*Publishers Weekly*

INTENSIVE CARE

"Shockingly believable . . . Intensive Care chronicles the voyage of an idealistic nursing student through the gritty realities of practice . . . with humor and a fine eye for detail."
—*The Washington Post*

"Compelling reading."
—*New York Daily News*

"Vivid . . . hard to put down . . . No one is spared her sharp lance. Nor does she spare herself."
—*St. Louis Post-Dispatch*

"Heron tells her story with a gripping, emotional intensity . . . With love and humor and vivid vignettes from her own life."
—*San Francisco Examiner*

CONDITION CRITICAL

"Critical care nurse Heron will make readers laugh and cry with this graphic, often shocking look at life in the trenches of a hospital in San Francisco . . . Heron writes with emotional intensity and sassy humor as she critiques the hospital's corner-cutting bureaucracy."
—*Publisher's Weekly*

"An uncompromising and often visionary sequel to her bestseller, *Intensive Care*. Fast-moving . . . passionate."
—*San Francisco Chronicle*

"In *CONDITION CRITICAL,* Heron frequently inspires laughter, tears, and awe through her vivid descriptions of a 'normal' workday. With keen sensibilities and wry expressiveness, she fleshes out brief patient vignettes in ways that haunt one's memory. . ."
—*Women's Magazine*

Printed in Great
Britain
by Amazon